Virgin Coconut Oil
Nature's Miracle Medicine

Dr. Bruce Fife

Piccadilly Books, Ltd.
Colorado Springs, CO

Every effort has been made to ensure that the information contained in this book is complete and accurate. However, neither the publisher nor the author is engaged in rendering professional advice or services to the individual reader. The ideas, procedures, and suggestions contained in this book are not intended as a substitute for consulting with your physician. All matters regarding your health require medical supervision. Neither the author nor the publisher shall be liable or responsible for any loss of damage allegedly arising from any information or suggestion in this book.

Piccadilly Books, Ltd.
P.O. Box 25203
Colorado Springs, CO 80936, USA
info@piccadillybooks.com
www.piccadillybooks.com

Library of Congress Cataloging-in-Publication Data
Fife, Bruce, 1952-
    Virgin coconut oil : nature's miracle medicine / Bruce Fife.
        p.cm.
    Summary: "Describes many of the health benefits of virgin coconut oil"--Provided by publisher.
    Includes bibliographical references.
    ISBN-13: 978-0-941599-64-1 (0-941599-64-7)
    1. Coconut oil--Health aspects--Popular works. 2. Fatty acids in human nutrition--Popular works. I. Title.
    QP752.F35F55   2006
    612.3'97--dc22

2006030938

Published in the USA
Printed in Canada

Contents

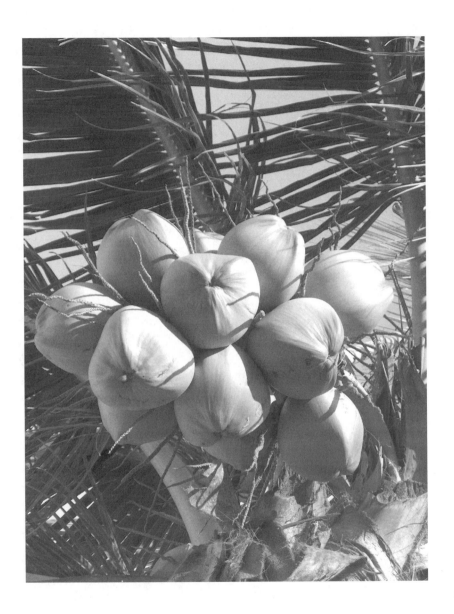

Chapter 1

A Miracle Oil

The auditorium was filled to capacity. "Where is he?" people were whispering as they glanced around the room. "Has Tony arrived yet?" someone asked. Tony was a special guest speaker at the symposium "Why Coconut Cures," held in the city of Manila, in the Philippines. In attendance were several hundred coconut enthusiasts, including physicians, scientists, and government officials. Also in attendance was one of Tony's doctors, Dr. Conrado Dayrit, a professor of pharmacology at the University of the Philippines and a former president of the National Academy of Science and Technology. You see, Tony is an AIDS survivor. He was at the symposium to tell the incredible story of his return from the dead.

"You don't know how hard it is for one to have an illness that others find repulsive," he told the audience, "I had wanted to shut myself inside my room and just wait for my time to die."

Tony was infected with HIV while working in the Middle East a few years earlier. When he returned home to the Philippines he was diagnosed with full blown AIDS. At this time Tony was in terrible shape. He was losing weight, had repeated bouts of vomiting and diarrhea, accompanied by a fever and persistent cough. Secondary infections encompassed his entire body. He had pneumonia, oral candidiasis, and chronic fatigue syndrome. He was so exhausted that he could hardly pull himself out of bed. His skin was covered with infections from head to toe. Everywhere his skin was flaking, cracking, and bleeding. His hair was falling out in clumps; he looked so bad he wore a wig to hide the bald spots and oozing sores in his scalp. The doctors didn't expect him to live much longer. "I felt like a candle that was starting to flicker and die," he said.

Unable to afford medication, he sought help from the Department of Health. He was referred to Dr. Conrado Dayrit. Dr. Dayrit had participated in a landmark HIV study a few years earlier. In this study, HIV infected patients were given the equivalent of 3.5 tablespoons of coconut oil a day. Because the patients couldn't afford medications they received no additional treatment. After three months, 60 percent of the patients were showing signs of improvement, a clear indication that the coconut oil treatment was working. Normally, without treatment those with HIV gradually get worse. Although numerous laboratory experiments had previously shown that coconut oil possessed antiviral properties that could knock out HIV, this was the first clinical study to verify these findings.

Dr. Dayrit instructed Tony to consume 6 tablespoons of coconut oil daily and apply additional coconut oil over the infections on his skin. Over the next several months when he would go back to the clinic for his periodic checkups the medical staff were amazed at his progress. They couldn't believe that he was improving more with the coconut oil than he had with the antiviral medications.

I met Tony for the first time at the conference. I was also one of the speakers. It was less than nine months since Tony had begun his coconut oil therapy. In this time his skin had completely cleared up. His hair had grown back, so that he no longer needed the wig. All of his secondary infections were gone. He got his energy back and he got his life back. You couldn't tell by looking at him that just a few months earlier he was literally on his death bed dying from AIDS.

Now, Tony may never be completely free from the AIDS virus. It will probably remain with him for life, but with regular use of coconut oil he is able to live a relatively normal life and enjoy a level of health much like everyone else.

Less than nine months after starting the coconut oil therapy, Tony stood before the audience to tell his story for the first time. "HIV virus has not been curable until now," he said. "The antiretrovirals cannot control the infection, which is why a lot of my friends died. Doctors

6

cannot predict how long I will live. When I was diagnosed, my doctors told me I wouldn't live another three months. Well, here I am now. I'm still standing."

In the Philippines coconut oil is called the "drugstore in a bottle" because this single oil can be used for so many purposes. It makes an excellent cooking oil and can be used for all types of frying or baking. It is recommended for those who have digestive problems or gallbladder disease because it is easy to digest. It improves the health of the digestive tract and is useful in treating conditions associated with irritable bowel syndrome such as Crohn's disease and colitis. It improves the absorption of vitamins and minerals and, therefore, is recommended for use in the treatment of malnutrition and certain nutritional deficiencies. It possesses potent anticancer properties and can be used in cancer treatment. It helps balance blood sugar and can be beneficial in reversing many of the symptoms associated with diabetes and hypoglycemia. It is a low-calorie fat that can aid in weight loss and weight management. Topically it makes an excellent moisturizer and skin rejuvenator. Perhaps the most incredible characteristics of coconut oil are its antibacterial, antiviral, and antifungal properties. It is because of these properties that Tony was able to eliminate all of his secondary bacterial, viral, and fungal infections and reduce his HIV load. For these reasons, coconut oil has been called the "healthiest oil on earth."

Coconut Oil is Unique

Coconut oil didn't always have such a good reputation. For many years coconut oil was considered one of the worst fats around. Indeed even today there are many misinformed people who believe that coconut oil is an "artery-clogging" saturated fat.

Over the past few decades saturated fats in general have been scrutinized because of their tendency to raise blood cholesterol. *All* saturated fats were considered bad and all were condemned by the media and health care professionals. Coconut oil with its high saturated fat content was blindly criticized along with the others. What people, including most health care professionals, didn't realize at the time was that there are many different types of saturated fat. Each of these saturated fats have a different effect on the body, some raise cholesterol,

7

some don't, and some, like those found in coconut oil, actually protect against heart disease. It wasn't until recently that health care professionals began to realize the differences among the saturated fats.

The type of saturated fat in coconut oil is unique. It is not like the saturated fats found in meats or even other vegetable oils. Coconut oil is composed of a special group of fat molecules known as medium-chain fatty acids (MCFA). Most all other fats in our diet, both saturated and unsaturated, are composed of long-chain fatty acids (LCFA). The primary difference between medium-chain fatty acids and long-chain fatty acids is the size of the molecule. As the name implies, MCFA are shorter or smaller than LCFA. The size of the molecule is extremely important because our bodies respond to and process each fat differently depending on its size. Therefore, the effects of MCFA in coconut oil are distinctly different from LCFA more commonly found in the diet. It is the MCFA in coconut oil that distinguishes it from all other oils and gives it its incredible healing properties.

The Proof

At first, some people are skeptical that coconut oil has all of the benefits I talk about. I can back up each claim with published medical studies. I've written several books on coconut and in these books I do include hundreds of references to studies so that readers can look them up and see for themselves. Although I do make reference to a few studies in this book my purpose here is not to overwhelm you with scientific proof but to simply present the facts.

Because this book is meant to be an introduction to the health aspects of coconut oil, I have kept technical information to a bare minimum and focused more on case histories and personal experiences. The real measure of the worth of a product is not found in laboratory measurements, but in how well it works in real life. Studies are good to have, but actual case histories reveal what happens in real life to real people in the real world. In this book you will find many such examples.

If you're looking for the science and chemistry behind coconut oil go to my website at www.coconutresearchcenter.org. Or better yet, read some of my other books on coconut (see pages 91-93). They present the science of coconut oil in simple terms so that even those with little scientific background can easily understand.

If you want proof of the value of coconut oil all you have to do is try it. You can prove it for yourself simply by using it. The primarily reason why coconut oil is rapidly growing in popularity is because it works! If it didn't work that would be the end of it and nobody would use it. But coconut oil's popularity is rapidly growing throughout the world. Let me share with you testimonies from a couple of satisfied users.

I started using coconut oil about six weeks ago and am delighted with the results. I am especially happy with this "discovery" because I actually grew up using coconut oil—I am a native of Guyana, South America, and we were always told, "A coconut a day keeps the doctor away." However, like so many people was later duped into believing that this miracle oil is unhealthy. Now I am so enthusiastic that I want to tell the whole world!
Sharon Maas

Those who begin using coconut oil regularly may notice improvements and changes in many aspects of their health as noted by the following individual.

I am a health professional and therefore not surprisingly, I was abashed when I would see books about coconut oil. Until my own health problems began. My thyroid levels were swinging around, but not really high enough to be treated by most allopathic doctors. I felt awful. My hair was falling out, my skin was so dry it itched and cracked, my cholesterol was up and so was my weight, ever so slowly with every passing month. In addition, my coworkers were amazed at how I could function when I am constantly sick and on antibiotics. I was a mess at a fairly young age.

I did some of my own research and kept coming up with coconut oil. Then I found your website (Coconut Research Center) and became more convinced as I accessed the journals presented. I felt like what was I to lose? Here is what happened after taking coconut oil for several months:

1) Weight has stopped increasing, it is starting to drop because I no longer crave sweets or simple carbs and have a massive surge of energy which allows me to be more active.

2) Cholesterol dropped, HDL [the good cholesterol] went WAY up (from 30's to almost 60).

3) My skin is beautiful! I was having rosacea, now it is smooth and clear. My legs feel as if I am a teenager they are so smooth. I even put coconut oil around my eyes as a moisturizer. I love feeling my legs, it is almost as if I have made a discovery. I cannot believe at my age my skin can be so soft and supple. It's almost like having a flashback to my teenage years!

4) I am not bloated anymore; my stomach not distended and my feet not hurting from not fitting in my shoes at the end of the day.

5) I feel so much more energetic, as if I was 10 years younger.

6) My hair is beautiful and silky and not falling out.

7) I am hardly ever sick anymore. When I or my kids are coming down with something, we up the coconut oil. We are better within a day.

8) My daughter was born with such extreme eczema, she was constantly itching, even had patches of scabs on her body and scalp. I have spent hundreds of dollars on expensive prescription steroid creams, which after a few years, stopped working. The doctor laughed at me when I mentioned coconut oil. The proof is in the fact that my daughter's skin is beautiful and flawless now, no itchy bumps, just beautiful baby skin. Even though she doesn't like the taste of coconut oil in her food she will eat it when I remind her of her skin problems. (She also is a very healthy weight.)

9) No more monthly yeast infections.

10) Wounds heal very quickly when coconut oil is applied. It's almost like magic.

11) My TSH levels are way down into the normal range (not even subclinical hypothyroid anymore). WOW! The first time in over 6 years!

It took quite a long time before I noticed these changes (several months). At first I gained weight and was very depressed by it all. I stuck with it. The health changes have been remarkable. Simply remarkable. Coconut oil has changed my life. The only sad part is, when I mention this to my colleagues or friends, I still get glazed-over looks of disinterest and disbelief, or outright gasps of horror with a refusal to listen to anymore of it.

Virgin Coconut Oil

The focus of this book is virgin coconut oil. What is virgin coconut oil and how is it different from other forms of coconut oil? There are basically two types of coconut oil: virgin coconut oil (VCO) and refined, bleached, and deodorized (RBD) coconut oil. The difference in the two is the way they are processed.

The term "virgin" is used to signify that the oil is pure and unadulterated, essentially the way nature made it, with as little processing as possible. Virgin coconut oil is extracted from *fresh* coconuts. To avoid contamination or poor quality, only the highest quality and freshest coconuts are used. Generally little or no heat is involved and absolutely no chemicals are used. The oil is as close as possible to the way nature made it with all its nutrients intact. As a consequence, virgin coconut oil maintains a mild coconut aroma and flavor. Since the oil is extracted from the white (colorless) meat of the coconut, good quality virgin coconut oil will be colorless. This is considered the highest quality and healthiest form of coconut oil. Virgin coconut oil that has been heated to excessive temperatures, as some are, will have a slight yellow appearance and perhaps a stronger flavor.

RBD oil, as the name implies, has undergone extensive refining, bleaching, and deodorizing. Unlike virgin coconut oil, RBD oil is made from *copra*. Copra is dried whole coconut. The quality of the coconut used to make copra varies. Fresh and old, damaged and undamaged nuts alike are used. Coconuts are cracked open and the meat is dried, usually by the sun, although ovens may also be used. Open coconuts are left in the sun exposed to the elements for days and even weeks before they are processed further. Consequently, the copra contains an appreciable amount of bacteria and mold. During the refining process the oil is sterilized and the contaminants are removed. Sometimes chemical agents are used in order to extract the greatest amount of oil from the meat and remove all contaminants. In the process everything is removed from the oil including all color, taste, and smell. The result is a colorless, tasteless, odorless oil.

RBD oil varies in purity and grade. A completely refined, bleached, and deodorized oil will be totally colorless, tasteless, and odorless. A less refined, lower grade RBD oil may have a slight yellow color and a mild taste. Oils that are even less fully refined will be a darker yellow and have a strong flavor. The flavor will not be like that of fresh coconut or virgin coconut oil. It will have a musty or chemical taste. The yellow color comes from residual contaminants that were not removed or from the excessive use of heat during processing. This is the lowest grade of coconut oil and is used most often in soaps and body lotions. Sometimes it is sold as cooking oil. It is not harmful to eat, but it doesn't taste as good as the other grades.

Both virgin and RBD coconut oils contain the beneficial MCFA that make coconut oil unique and beneficial. You can get much of the same benefit from eating RBD coconut oil as you do from virgin coconut oil. Virgin coconut oil, however, has an added benefit. Since it has gone through less processing it retains most of the phytonutrients that are naturally found in the raw, unprocessed coconut oil. This includes antioxidants and phytosterols which are known to have heart protective, anticancer, and other health promoting properties. These phytonutrients have been stripped from RBD coconut oil during processing.

Virgin coconut oil is considered a premium quality health food. Good quality virgin coconut oil has a mild pleasant taste that is so good it can be eaten by the spoonful. It can be used in cooking and food preparation without imparting a strong coconut flavor. Virgin coconut oil should not have a strong flavor. If it does then it may be poorly processed or it may actually be a low quality RBD oil. The highest quality oils are colorless with a mild aroma and pleasant flavor.

In addition to color and taste another way you can identify a poor quality coconut oil or oil that is going rancid is how it feels in the throat. A poor quality oil will produce a slight burning sensation or irritation in the back of the throat. This is often referred to as a "catch in the throat." This sensation is most noticeable when the oil is taken by itself rather than with food. A good quality virgin coconut oil will not produce this sensation.

One of the characteristics of all types of coconut oil whether it is virgin or not is its high melting point. Coconut oil melts at 76 degrees F (24 C). Above this temperature it is a clear liquid. Below this temperature it solidifies and becomes a white solid. People not aware of this characteristic have purchased coconut oil as a colorless liquid and brought it home and after a few days to their surprise it has transformed into a hard white solid. The first thought is that the oil has gone rancid or something else is wrong with it. This is not so. This is just a characteristic of the oil. You can use it hard or soft. All oils have a melting point. If you put butter in the refrigerator it turns solid. But if you take it out on a hot day it melts into a puddle. Likewise, olive oil will become solid in the refrigerator, but at room temperature it remains liquid.

Virgin coconut oil is generally sold in bottles, much like any cooking oil. Because the oil hardens in cool temperatures the bottles normally have wide mouths for easy access. When hardened, it can be easily scooped out with a spoon or knife.

In addition to using virgin coconut oil for cooking and baking many people take it as a dietary supplement. Generally they take it by the spoonful. A good quality virgin coconut oil tastes good and most people don't have a problem taking it this way. If you can't stand the taste of the oil then you are probably using a poor quality oil and need to change brands.

Chapter 2

Coconut Oil is Good for Your Heart

The biggest fear people have about eating coconut oil is the idea that it is bad for the heart. You can rest assured that coconut oil will not harm your heart. Coconut oil is heart healthy and will help protect you from heart disease.

When I travel to coconut growing regions of the world and talk to the people, they tell me how their parents and grandparents ate coconuts and coconut oil every day of their lives and lived to ripe old ages without experiencing heart disease. Studies confirm this. Research has shown that those people who rely on coconut as the primary source of fat in their diets have a remarkably low rate of heart disease. In fact, those people who eat the most coconut oil have the lowest heart disease rates in the world.

For example, in a survey of heart disease death rates of 36 countries the lowest was the Philippines.[1] The countries in the survey included most all the those in Eastern and Western Europe and North America and many in Latin America and Asia. The Philippines was the only coconut consuming country in the list. The Philippines is the world's largest coconut oil producer and consumer. In the survey Russia had the highest heart disease death rate at 1802 per 100,000 people. Japan had the second lowest at 548 per 100,000. Japan is known for its overall good health and longevity, yet the heart disease death rate in the

---

1. Fife, B. *Coconut Cures: Preventing and Treating Common Health Problems with Coconut*. Colorado Springs, CO: Piccadilly Books, 2005.

Philippines was a mere 120 per 100,000 – more than 4.5 times *less* than that of Japan! The United States with an advanced medical system and the highest health care costs in the world has a heart disease death rate 7 times greater than that of the Philippines. If coconut oil is so bad for the heart why is heart disease so much lower in coconut eating countries?

Most countries in the world have adopted western medicine and dietary practices and recommendations. Even most countries in the coconut growing regions of the world have moved away from using coconut oil due to a fear of saturated fat. As these people have switched from the use of coconut oil to processed vegetable oils and margarines the heart disease rates have *risen*, not declined as expected. For this reason, heart disease is on the rise worldwide. Studies show that populations that still rely on coconut oil as their primary source of fat have a *complete absence of heart disease*.[2, 3, 4] That's right. In those areas of the world where people rely heavily on coconut oil, heart disease virtually does not exist. Researchers have found that people in these populations can live into their 90s yet are still completely free from all signs of heart disease.[5] It appears that not only is coconut oil not harmful, but actually protects against heart disease.

The Good and Bad Cholesterol
There are different types of cholesterol circulating in our blood. In general, they are referred to as the "good" and the "bad" cholesterol. The bad cholesterol, otherwise known as *LDL cholesterol*, gets its

2. Lindeberg, S., et al. Cardiovascular risk factors in a Melanesian population apparently free from stroke and ischaemic heart disease; the Kitava study. *J Intern Med* 1994;236:331-340.
3. Mendis, S. Coronary heart disease and coronary risk profile in a primitive population. *Trop Geogr Med* 1991;43:199-202.
4. Prior, I.A.M. et al Cholesterol, coconuts, and diet on Polynesian atolls: a natural experiment: the Pukapuka and Tokelau Island studies. *Am J Clin Nutr* 1981;34:1552.
5. Lindeberg, S. and Lundh, B.A. Apparent absence of stroke and ischaemic heart disease in a traditional Melanesian island: a clinical study in Kitava. *J Intern Med* 1993;233:269-275.

notoriety from the fact that it transports cholesterol throughout the body. It therefore, carries the cholesterol that might possibly become trapped in artery walls and clog the arteries. *HDL cholesterol* is considered the good guy because it brings cholesterol back to the liver for reprocessing and possible elimination from the body. HDL cholesterol is believed to protect against heart disease and the more you have the better. Therefore, high HDL cholesterol values reduce risk of heart disease.

When people talk about blood cholesterol they generally refer only to *total* cholesterol. When total cholesterol is measured it includes both LDL (bad) and HDL (good) cholesterol so you don't know how much you have of each. The average person has a total cholesterol reading of about 200 mg/dl. For many years values above this were considered high and values below that were considered low, thus indicating high and low risk for heart disease. A major problem with this method of judging risk was that it doesn't work very well. Nearly half of all those people who die of heart attacks have normal to below normal *total* cholesterol levels.

The Cholesterol Ratio

A far more accurate indicator of heart disease risk is the *cholesterol ratio* (total cholesterol/HDL). The cholesterol ratio takes into account the amount of HDL (good) cholesterol that is in the total, thus getting a much better indication of heart disease risk.

Researchers have determined that a cholesterol ratio of 5.0 is average or normal. A ratio above 5.0 indicates an increased risk of heart disease and below 5.0 a reduction in risk. A ratio of 3.2 or less is considered optimal or the lowest risk.

Although *total* cholesterol has proven to be an unreliable indicator of heart disease risk, it is the value that people still most often refer to when they get blood work done. The overemphasis on total cholesterol is perpetuated by the pharmaceutical industry as a means to sell cholesterol-lowering drugs. For this reason, there is a lot of confusion about cholesterol values.

Let's look at an example. If you have a total cholesterol reading of 240 mg/dl, this would be considered high because it is over 200. You would be told that you are at high risk for heart disease. However, if your HDL (good) cholesterol was 75 mg/dl, your cholesterol ratio would be 3.2. This value is in the optimal range and you would have the lowest risk. Since the cholesterol ratio is a far more accurate indicator of heart disease risk, even though your total cholesterol may be high, your actual risk is very low.

The opposite can also happen. If you have a total cholesterol reading of 180 mg/dl, that would be said to indicate low risk. If, however, your HDL was only 32 mg/dl, your cholesterol ratio would be 5.6 mg/dl, which is in the *high risk* category! So a person with low total cholesterol can be at high risk and a person with high total cholesterol can be at low risk. You need to know the cholesterol ratio to find your true risk. This explains why so many people who die of heart disease have normal or below normal total cholesterol levels and why many people with high total cholesterol levels live long lives without experiencing heart problems.

Now there are people who have both high total cholesterol and a high cholesterol ratio and people who have both low total cholesterol and a low cholesterol ratio. My point is this, if you only look at your total cholesterol value, as most people tend to do, you can come to a completely wrong conclusion as to heart disease risk. To accurately judge heart disease risk from cholesterol values you must use the cholesterol ratio, not total cholesterol.

Coconut Oil and Cholesterol

One of the biggest misconceptions about coconut oil is that it is high in cholesterol. This is completely false. Coconut oil contains absolutely no cholesterol whatsoever. Cholesterol is found *only* in animal fats. Coconut oil comes from a plant so it is cholesterol-free.

Another misconception is that coconut oil raises blood cholesterol and thus contributes to heart disease. The idea that all saturated fats raise cholesterol is a gross oversimplification. All saturated fats do not raise cholesterol. Although the MCFA in coconut oil are saturated they are heart friendly and help to protect against heart disease.

Coconut oil does *not* have a harmful effect on cholesterol levels. Read that last sentence over again because it is very important for you to understand. Coconut oil is heart friendly, more so than probably any other dietary fat.

When coconut oil is added into the diet the effects on cholesterol levels vary from individual to individual. Some people see little change while others experience dramatic changes as noted in the following examples.

I had some concerns of the effects of virgin coconut oil (I thought it may bring up my chol/trigs levels.) After a month of use—2 tablespoons a day and after a lipid panel evaluation, no change in these values. They stayed the same as the blood work one year ago had indicated. The proof is in black and white (the lab results).

Ray L.

You may be interested to know that since taking the oil for two and a half years my cholesterol has dropped from the danger level, my triglycerides are right down, I have stopped taking heart tablets (now 113 over 73), lost 24 kgs (53 lbs), and hair growth and color turning back to original. My wife has lost 24 kgs and my daughter 14 kgs (31 lbs).

RJ

Just got back from the doctor's office and my total cholesterol went from 260 to 180. My doctor was so happy. I've been going to her for over 15 years and dreaded every time I got the blood test, it was always the same thing—a lecture.

I had always used olive oil for years but started using coconut oil for most of our cooking (olive oil occasionally). I also made my own version of coconut treats using coconut oil and bitter chocolate with shredded coconut and stevia, vanilla, coconut cream, real salt mixed and spooned onto wax paper in the shape of haystacks (coconut candies). Could do the same with nuts but I really like coconut and had my tablespoons of oil this way. Must have done something right, it worked!...Did I also mention my triglycerides went from 187 to 109?

SA

Awhile back I went to the doctor for a routine yearly physical. I am 51 years old about 6 feet 1 inch and on that date 221 pounds. Blood work revealed a triglyceride level of 400, total cholesterol of 237, and HDL of 40. I was shocked. I started to look around on the Internet to find out what I might do to better my situation and somewhere I read about the virtues of coconut products. This struck me as odd because I had always heard about how bad coconut and other tropical oils were and somewhere along the way I found and purchased your book The Coconut Oil Miracle *which has been a revelation to me. Through cutting out most all refined sugars, reducing the amount of white potatoes, and bread products made with bleached white flours, and replacing all hydrogenated cooking oils and margarine with coconut oil, I have achieved some astonishing results. After following these new guidelines for five or six weeks I went in for another blood draw. Weight is now at 197 pounds, triglycerides 85, total cholesterol 145, and HDL 44. Thank you very much for your research and your perseverance to get out the truth about coconut products when it wasn't and probably still isn't a popular thing to do.*
    Jeff C.

    For many years measuring cholesterol levels has been a convenient tool for doctors to gauge heart disease risk. In the past the only cholesterol measurement recorded was total cholesterol. Over time researchers discovered that some forms of cholesterol (HDL) were actually good for you and reduced the risk of heart disease. This confused the issue tremendously.
    Up to this time numerous studies had been done to measure cholesterol values after people had eaten different types of oils. It was discovered that polyunsaturated vegetable oils, such as soybean, safflower, and corn oils reduced total cholesterol better than coconut oil. This was interpreted to mean that polyunsaturated vegetables oils protect against heart disease while coconut oil didn't. The problem with these studies is that they only measured total cholesterol, while ignoring HDL (good) cholesterol.
    New studies were performed to measure the different fractions of cholesterol and calculate the cholesterol ratios. An interesting

discovery was made. Coconut oil was found to increase HDL cholesterol relative to LDL and total cholesterol. Although most vegetable oils reduce *total* cholesterol more than coconut oil does, coconut oil *improves* the cholesterol ratio more than any other oil! Therefore, based on the cholesterol ratio, *coconut oil protects against heart disease better than any other oil.*

There was a very interesting study done in Sri Lanka where coconut oil is commonly used.[6] Cholesterol levels were measured in subjects whose normal diet included coconut oil. Subjects were then given corn oil, a polyunsaturated vegetable oil, to replace the coconut oil in their diets. After several weeks their cholesterol values were again measured. This is what they discovered. When these people switched from using coconut oil to corn oil their total cholesterol decreased on average from 179.6 to 146.0 mg/dl. Their LDL (bad) cholesterol also decreased on average from 131.6 to 100.3 mg/dl. Both of these changes are considered good, and if taken by themselves, would suggest that corn oil is superior to coconut oil in protecting against heart disease.

However, when the HDL (good) cholesterol values were also taken into account the picture completely changed. The HDL cholesterol in the subjects also decreased from 43.4 to 25.4 mg/dl, which is not good. The cholesterol ratio increased from 4.14 to 5.75, which definitely is not good. Remember that a cholesterol ratio of 5.0 is average. When these people were eating coconut oil their cholesterol ratio was 4.14, which indicates low risk. When they switched to corn oil, a supposedly heart friendly polyunsaturated oil, their cholesterol ratio jumped to an average of 5.75. This is in the high risk category. So even though corn oil lowered total cholesterol, it increased the cholesterol ratio and, therefore, increased the risk of heart disease as compared to coconut oil. So according to this study coconut oil protects against heart disease, while corn oil promotes it.

I have found that when people add coconut oil into their diets their total cholesterol may rise slightly or fall slightly, but in either case their

---

6. Mendis, S., et al. The effects of replacing coconut oil with corn oil on human serum lipid profiles and platelet derived factors active in atherogenesis. *Nutrition Reports International* Oct. 1989;40(4).

HDL (good) cholesterol increases, thus lowering their cholesterol ratio and lowering their risk of heart disease.

Sometimes people will become alarmed when after using coconut oil for a time they find that their total cholesterol has increased. Why did their total cholesterol increase? I explain to them that it is because their HDL (good) cholesterol has increased, therefore, their total cholesterol is higher. Remember, total cholesterol alone is not a good indicator of heart disease risk. Nowadays both total and HDL values are commonly measured at the same time. Comparing your old values, you can calculate the cholesterol ratio before using coconut oil and afterwards. In most every case the cholesterol ratio improves. Thus coconut oil has reduced the risk of heart disease.

Here is an actual case. A lady had been using coconut oil for three years. When she had blood work done her total cholesterol was measured at 268. Normally this is considered very high. However, her HDL was measured at 149, giving her a cholesterol ratio of only 1.8! This is an incredibly low value indicating an extremely low risk for heart disease.

Here's another example. A woman had a family history of high cholesterol. Family members had total cholesterol readings in excess of 400 mg/dl. After adding coconut oil into her diet her total cholesterol rose from 336 to 376 mg/dl. Ordinarily this is considered very high. However, her HDL (good) cholesterol nearly doubled from 65 to 120 mg/dl. Her cholesterol ratio dropped from a high risk value of 5.2 mg/dl to a low risk value of 3.1 mg/dl, which is within the optimal range. Although she had a very high total cholesterol reading, her true risk was very low. Her blood pressure was optimal at 110/60.

Virgin coconut oil appears to have a balancing effect on blood fats. In some people it decreases total cholesterol while in others it increases it. In either case, however, the cholesterol ratio always improves, thus reducing risk of heart disease.

Virgin coconut oil (VCO) intake in substantial amounts keeps cholesterol low, between 170 and 200 ml/dl, by promoting the conversion of cholesterol into pregnenolone to be utilized in the production of adrenal and sex hormones. VCO's cholesterol-lowering effect is a regulatory action since it can also beneficially

raise cholesterol when it is too low for the body's needs, thus maintaining the healthy ratio between low density lipoprotein-cholesterol and high density lipoprotein-cholesterol (HDL).
Conrado Dayrit, MD, Cardiologist

In some people coconut oil will have very little effect on their total cholesterol. Total cholesterol may remain essentially unchanged. However, that doesn't mean nothing has happened. Coconut oil increases HDL so even though total cholesterol may not change much *the cholesterol ratio improves* and, consequently, heart disease risk drops.

In most every case that I've seen when people start using coconut oil their cholesterol ratio decreases. In those rare occasions where the cholesterol ratio has not improved, the problem has been tracked to dietary factors unrelated to coconut oil and once these factors have been adjusted the cholesterol ratio improves. Take the following example.

A woman who had been using coconut for about a year contacted me. She was worried and confused. She had just received results from her most recent cholesterol test. While taking the coconut oil her cholesterol levels had increased. She wanted answers. Why were her numbers so different from those of others?

She had her cholesterol levels measured a year before she began to use coconut oil. Her total cholesterol at that time was 165, HDL 60, LDL 80 and her cholesterol ratio was an incredibly low 2.75, indicating very low risk for heart disease. For the past 20 years her cholesterol values had not varied by more than 5 or 10 mg/dl. Her most recent test showed that all of her cholesterol levels had increased significantly: total cholesterol 236, HDL 82, and LDL 132. Her cholesterol ratio also increased to 2.88.

I explained to her that even though her cholesterol ratio increased slightly, 2.88 still indicates extremely low risk. It didn't help. She was still worried, especially since her total cholesterol had increased so dramatically from 165 to 236.

We looked at her diet. Nothing in her diet had changed over the past year except to add coconut oil. She ate absolutely no meat or dairy products. She was a complete vegan and had been so for many years. The only animal product she ate was a fish oil dietary supplement. I mentioned that fish oil may elevate cholesterol levels.

22

She stopped using the fish oil supplements for three weeks and then got another blood test. To her surprise her total cholesterol fell 57 mg/dl, from 236 to 179. HDL fell a bit to 70, and her LDL fell much more—from 132 to 85. Her cholesterol ratio was now 2.56, which was lower than it was a year ago, indicating that the coconut oil had improved her cholesterol profile. Simply eliminating a dietary supplement had a significant impact on her cholesterol values.

Studies have consistently shown that coconut oil increases HDL and improves the cholesterol ratio. While coconut oil does not reduce *total* cholesterol as effectively as polyunsaturated oils do, it has a greater effect on HDL. When HDL and cholesterol ratio values are evaluated, it is seen that coconut oil reduces risk of heart disease more than fish oil or soybean, canola, safflower, corn or any other vegetable oil typically recommended as "heart healthy." Therefore, judging from cholesterol values, coconut oil protects against heart disease better than any other oil. It is the ultimate "heart friendly" dietary oil.

High Blood Pressure

Another risk factor for heart disease that is even more significant than cholesterol is blood pressure. Elevated blood pressure is not only associated with an increased risk of heart disease but evidence shows it can even cause it. Reducing high blood pressure is an important step in lowering the risk of heart disease.

Blood pressure is simply the force exerted by the blood being pumped through the blood vessels. As blood pressure increases, the force acting on the artery walls increases, causing stress that can cause minute rips or tears in the lining of the artery wall. This causes inflammation, blood clotting, and the deposition of fat and scar tissue at the site of injury. If blood pressure is not reduced, the injury remains under stress and inflammation and fat and protein deposition continues. This material, known as plaque, gradually narrows the artery canal. If the canal becomes obstructed with plaque a heart attack or stroke may result. Therefore, keeping blood pressure within normal limits is vitally important to your health.

Blood pressure is expressed as two numbers, one on top of the other. Normal average blood pressure is indicated as 120/80. The top

23

number indicates the pressure when the heart is contracting and actively pumping the blood. The lower number is the pressure between beats when the heart is relaxed. High blood pressure is usually defined as a resting blood pressure greater than 140/90. Readings above 130/80 are considered elevated and still within normal but indicate a risk for developing high blood pressure.

The harder it is to pump blood through the arteries the greater the stress is on the heart. Excessive stress can overwork the heart promoting heart failure. Therefore, lower blood pressure is generally healthier for the heart. Although 120/80 is regarded as normal, values somewhat below this are even better.

Many people who have high blood pressure have reported that when they add coconut oil into their diets their blood pressure comes down.

I began using coconut oil 11 days ago. I went to the doctor's office the Friday before and my blood pressure was 169/94, now my blood pressure is 112/68. Here are a few other changes I have noticed, hair (stopped breaking), skin (not dry and flakey). I take 1 tablespoon in hot tea every morning and another 1 tablespoon at lunch on my salad, and add 1-2 tablespoons in my dinner meal. Did I tell you how much energy I have now?
Ella

Three years ago I was taking heart tablets with a blood pressure of 165 over 90, last year I stopped taking them as the coconut oil seemed to have reduced the pressure. The reading remained between 116/62 to 121/74. Well five weeks ago I ran out of virgin coconut oil and I thought that I'll just hang on until we start making it ourselves. Two weeks later after a bit of a weekend, I could feel there was something wrong and I took my blood pressure and found that it had jumped to 161/99. I had a friend that I had given some oil to and knew he was not consuming it, got it back and started consuming 60 ml a day... I took my reading every day and found the blood pressure slowly dropping every day and it is down at the moment at 121/74. This came as a bit of

24

a surprise to me, but somehow the coconut oil is keeping my blood pressure down.
Grant

Improved Circulation

Research has shown that MCFA in coconut oil have a stimulatory effect on metabolism. After a single meal containing MCFA, metabolism can rise by as much as 65 percent. As metabolism increases, blood flow also increases. This increase in circulation is often felt as an increase in energy and a rise in body temperature. Many people with chronic low temperatures report how using coconut oil increases their circulation and brings their temperatures back up to normal or close to it.

Here are some typical responses.

My temperature was always low, about 97 degrees. After a few weeks of eating coconut oil it was up to normal.
CH

Coconut oil is fantastic. I have found that I can go longer between meals and my temps have risen to a normal 98.6, instead of 96.4, which has been typical for the last six years. And with the increase of temperature I have been effortlessly losing weight.
Roby

I have been taking virgin coconut oil for about two months, but only in the last week have I reached the recommended 3.5 tablespoons per day. The resultant rise in body temperature has been quite striking—it jumped from 96.2 to 97.1 in a 24 hour period and has stayed up there for over a week now.
Katy

I too experienced quite the increase in body temperature (taken first thing in the morning). It raised from low 97's to 98.4-98.8! I don't feel near as cold as I used to, my energy levels have come

back and much more stable. I don't feel the brain fogginess that I experienced, my hair is so soft and my nails are growing at a rapid rate! I absolutely love it.
Jen

Since taking the coconut oil on a daily basis, I no longer experience the sharp blood sugar level decreases around lunch and dinner times that caused irritability, poor concentration, tiredness and the desire to seek fatty foods and/or foods high in carbohydrates and proteins...Other noticeable health benefits I have noticed over the past 4 or 5 months is an improvement in my circulation (very noticeable over this winter) and improved skin complexion.
LW

Blood carries oxygen and nutrients throughout the body. When circulation is restricted problems can arise. Every cell and organ in your body needs a continual supply of oxygen in order to function. Without a continuous source of oxygen our cells suffocate and die. Even a partial restriction of blood flow can adversely affect the body. As noted by Jen above, improving her circulation by using coconut oil helped to bring more oxygen to her brain, thus clearing her brain fog. It also increased her energy levels and helped the growth of her hair and nails. LW reported improvement in concentration, more energy, and better blood sugar control.

Good circulation is not only important for overall health but is vital for the health of your heart. In fact, it is a restriction in blood flow that causes heart attacks. If the flow of blood in the arteries feeding the heart is blocked or restricted, the heart cannot get the oxygen it needs. The heart muscle begins to die. The result is a heart attack. So maintaining good circulation is vital to the heart. Coconut oil improves blood circulation and, therefore, aids in protecting against heart attacks.

Coconut Oil Protects the Heart

Coconut oil improves cholesterol values, helps lower elevated blood pressure, and enhances blood circulation, all of which indicate the

26

protective nature of coconut oil on the heart. This is evidenced by the many cultures throughout the world that rely heavily on the use of coconuts and coconut oil and have a remarkably low incidence of heart disease. Judging from the evidence, if you want to prevent a heart attack you should be using coconut oil.

Not everyone knows about the health benefits of coconut. Many think of it as just another saturated fat that is bad for the heart. You can't blame them, that's what they've heard for years. They're only speaking out of ignorance. They have yet to learn about the heart protective nature of coconut oil and all of its health benefits. You can help educate them by sharing this book with them.

Chapter 3

Nature's Amazing Germ Fighter

Virgin coconut oil is becoming recognized as the healthiest of all dietary oils. What makes it so healthy are medium-chain fatty acids (MCFA).

All fats and oils are composed of fat molecules known as fatty acids. There are many different types of fatty acids, but they all can be classified into three basic categories: short-chain fatty acids (SCFA), medium-chain fatty acids (MCFA), and long-chain fatty acids (LCFA). Almost all of the fats in our diet consist of LCFA. Coconut oil is unique. It is compose predominately of MCFA.

The fatty acids in our foods, whether they are short, medium, or long, are in the form of triglycerides. Triglycerides are simply three fatty acids that are joined together. So you can have short-chain triglycerides (SCT), medium-chain triglycerides (MCT), or long-chain triglycerides (LCT). Coconut oil actually consists of MCT. When a fat is consumed, our bodies break the bonds that hold the triglycerides together releasing the individual fatty acids. It is only after the oil is consumed that the MCT transform into MCFA. This is important because MCFA can have a very powerful effect on our health.

One of the most remarkable effects of MCFA in coconut oil is their ability to prevent and even cure infectious illnesses.[7] So powerful are they that MCFA are currently being used in food processing to

7. Kabara, J.J. *The Pharmacological Effects of Lipids*. Champaign, IL: The American Oil Chemist's Society 1978.

protect foods from spoilage by bacteria and fungi. They are also included in dietary supplements and skin lotions to combat infections. Even some over-the-counter antibacterial, antiviral, and antifungal medications include MCFA as the active ingredient.

Like Mother's Milk

There are only a few foods that contain MCFA. Coconut oil is by far the best source. Palm kernel oil also contains a fair amount. The next best source is human breast milk. Breast milk contains about 4-9 percent MCFA, depending on the mother's diet. Mother Nature apparently sees the need for MCFA in the diet of newborn infants or they wouldn't be there. Researchers have studied the need for MCFA in human growth and development. They have discovered numerous benefits and for this reason coconut oil or MCT are routinely added to baby formulas.

One of the primary reasons why nature puts MCFA in breast milk is to protect the infant from infections. When a baby is born its immune system is still immature and the infant is very vulnerable to a world teaming with infectious organisms. Researchers have determined that it is due primarily to the presence of MCFA in breast milk that protects newborns from infections for the first few months of their lives.

Virgin coconut oil is immunoprotective in children, superior to vitamin C...Clinical studies show virgin coconut oil's significant role in pediatrics as a source of energy, an immune system booster, a local antiseptic, and an anti-inflammatory.

Arturo C. Ludan, MD
Pediatrician/gastroenterologist

Since the 1960s hundreds of published studies have demonstrated the effectiveness of MCFA in killing disease causing microorganisms. Research shows that MCFA in coconut oil are effective in destroying viruses that cause influenza, measles, herpes, mononucleosis, hepatitis C, and AIDS; bacteria which can cause stomach ulcers, throat infections, pneumonia, sinusitis, ear infections, rheumatic fever, gum disease, food poisoning, urinary tract infections, and gonorrhea; fungi and yeast which cause ringworm, athlete's food, toe and nail fungus, candida/yeast infections, and thrush; and parasites that can cause intestinal infections such as giardiasis.

While MCFA are deadly to harmful microorganisms, they are completely harmless to us. This has led scientists to postulate that MCFA could be useful as a treatment against infectious illnesses and as an additive to preserve food. Both coconut oil and purified MCFA are currently being utilized for these purposes.

We know that breast milk is effective in protecting newborns from infections. Coconut oil contains 10 times as much disease fighting MCFA as human breast milk. It, therefore, can be useful in not only preventing infectious disease, but curing them as well. Tony's story in Chapter 1 is a good example of this.

Protection from Disease

MCFA have been used in certain anti-fungal over-the-counter medications for many years. One of the most common conditions caused by fungal infections is the single-celled fungus (yeast) known as *Candida albicans*. Candida overgrowth often occurs around mucous membranes such as the mouth (thrush) or vagina (yeast infection). It can also affect the surface of the skin when the skin is kept in a moist environment (diaper rash). Systemic Candida infections can affect the entire digestive tract and can be very difficult to treat. Consuming coconut oil and making modifications to the diet can reduce or eliminate the infection.

I know another good use for coconut oil. I have recurrent vaginal yeast infections, one each month! Coconut oil has antifungal properties. I have tried others and am still looking for the right combo of herbals, but so far coconut oil has given me the most relief!
MR

I have been using coconut oil for over a year now and need I say it has made a tremendous change in my life over the course of this time! I am an endurance athlete and have also had major

30

Candida problems built up for many years from over carbohydrate/ sugar consumption that is now completely gone. I'm back to being in excellent health again!
Ronan

Another common fungus is tinea. There are many forms of tinea which can cause a variety of skin infections. Rubbing coconut oil on the infected skin can relieve the symptoms and get rid of the infection. Coconut oil is very effective in treating skin fungus as noted in the following examples.

We tried it on our feet, between the toes. It stops tinea (skin fungus). After wearing bikini liners on a monthly basis I find that this area can become itchy. So, after a shower I applied some carefully covering creases. It only took one application and the itch was gone. It's terrific! No more expensive antifungal creams required for this family. It works!
Sue

I am a believer from experience! One of the big problems with skin yeast and fungal infections is that clothing tends to absorb or else rub off the expensive medicine after application. This time I wasn't looking forward to applying the strong liquid prescription to it because the kind I have stings—big time—when it hits the red, angry, sore area of the yeast infection in the skin folds. I had some virgin coconut oil left in a small jar which I was using for smoothing on after a shower. I took that out and just slathered it on. Instantly the pain was soothed away and for the moment anyway, that was enough. By the end of the day I could tell that the coconut oil was doing more than just relieving the soreness. The rash was breaking up a little and there were some small clear areas where before it was just solid red soreness. I applied the coconut oil twice a day and in three-four days the whole area is mostly pink and clearing. And it isn't staining clothing either!
Beverly

I told my husband that coconut oil was antifungal and one time he started putting it on his athlete's food. He doesn't have a lot of trouble with it, but once in awhile he would put medicated cream on it. He was aghast when the coconut oil made his athlete's food completely stop bothering him.
Laura

I had a place in my ear where it would not quit itching. I don't know if it was a fungus, but on the inside of my ear it would get extremely itchy and it was like this for months. It would flake off on the inside (sounds gross, it wasn't that bad though) but I put some coconut oil on it and it went away overnight. I did not drop the oil way into my ear, but took a Q-tip with some oil on it and rubbed it on the outside and just right on the inside of my ear.
Jill

The MCFA in coconut oil are effective in killing many different types of bacteria that cause illness and disease. This is one of its purposes in mother's milk. You can say, in essences, it is nature's disinfectant.

I love this incredible virgin coconut oil. I had a hard lump behind my ear for over a month and since I couldn't see it, I went to my nice, but traditional western dermatologist. He told me it was a cyst and that he wanted to inject it with cortisone and if that didn't work that the plastic surgeon on staff should remove it. HA! I don't think so. I told him thank you but I just wanted his diagnosis and that I would try a home remedy first before any injection. I put virgin coconut oil on it before bed, woke up and it was half the size! By the 3rd day of virgin coconut oil it is barely a pinhead. The pain is gone and I am so happy.
Lisa

Coconut oil not only kills bacteria that cause minor illnesses but also some very serious ones as well. Bubonic plague is a highly contagious disease caused by a microscopic bacterium. It is transmitted to people by fleas from infected rats and other rodents. It is often called the *black death* because of the appearance of dark spots that develop from bleeding under the skin. The disease gained notoriety because at one time it caused severe epidemics throughout Europe and Asia. Outbreaks continue to occur in Asia and Africa with isolated cases turning up in all countries.

In his book *Nature the Healer,* author John Richter relates the following interesting experience. "When I was in Panama, I visited three different cases of black death, the plague they dread so down there. Black death is really a tropical affliction, since the cold air of the north seems to destroy the germs. In tropical countries coconuts are plentiful and very good. I got the patients I mentioned to drink coconut milk in quantities and they got well. This got the health officers of the hospitals interested and coconut milk is used for the cure of bubonic plague."

Most bacterial infections can be treated with antibiotics. Viruses are another matter. There are no antiviral medications that can effectively kill viruses. Antibiotics only kill bacteria. They are completely useless against viruses. They are sometimes prescribed by doctors in treating viruses, not because they do anything to the virus but because they might prevent secondary infections from opportunistic bacteria.

Scientists have yet to create an antiviral drug that is effective in killing viruses. All that antivirals can do is help reduce the severity of an infection. The body has to mount the attack to eventually rid itself of an invading virus. When you are infected by a virus there is not much the doctor can do for you. If he gives you medications they are to help relieve the discomfort of symptoms rather than fight the infection.

Nature, however, has provided us with a potent antiviral in the form of MCFA. Again the miracle of mother's milk and coconut oil come to the rescue. With coconut oil we now have an effective means by which to fight viral infections.

My husband had a bad sore on his hand. We thought it was cancer. It just wouldn't go away. I insisted he go to a dermatologist. He went and he was told, no cancer, something amiss in the blood and it had something to do with a viral problem. I started using coconut oil on his hand. Now mind you, he had had this on his hand for about two years. Within three weeks it went away!! It has never come back!
JL

One of the most common viral infections is the flu. When you get the flu the doctor can't do much for you. You've got to sit it out and let the body do its thing. Adding coconut oil into your diet may greatly reduce the symptoms and the duration of the illness. When you first start feeling the signs of the flu coming on I recommend that you take a spoonful of coconut oil every couple of hours until you feel better.

I was coming down with a sore throat and general aches and pains on Sunday/Monday and that "omg" feeling that I was going to be battling with feeling bad for a week or more. I was already treating myself with extra Vitamin C (which I have found very helpful through personal experience) and I take 4+Tbs virgin coconut oil a day anyway.

I just happened to be flicking through Bruce's Coconut Oil Miracle *book where he talks about curing flu symptoms with extra virgin coconut oil. So on Tuesday, I added an extra 2 tablespoons to my diet that day (making a total of more than 6 tablespoons) and by that evening, I suddenly realized that I didn't feel so bad any more! The next day (Wednesday) I also added in more virgin coconut oil than usual and today I basically feel completely well (perhaps a bit tired).*

Katy

There has been a nasty stomach virus going around the New York City area. I was hit with it on a Sunday mid-afternoon. I had two bowel "episodes" which made me know I had the virus, just like my brother and our mother and father. Later that day I took about two tablespoons of liquid virgin coconut oil and I also took some cider vinegar with water. For dinner, I had a sweet potato drenched in coconut oil.

I never had another episode. My friends and family had been telling me about how long the virus stayed with them—some for seven days or more. Mine only lasted for an afternoon. That evening I was back to normal.

I'm glad I've been finding out about all the incredible things coconut and coconut oil can do for you.

Vince S

I found myself leafing through Bruce Fife's book just before Christmas, and was
so fascinated that I walked out having bought the book and a jar of organic unrefined coconut oil. Immediately I started using it on my skin and added a small amount to my diet. On New Year's Eve I felt the onslaught of the flu....scratchy throat and fatigue....so I added more coconut oil to a soup I was making (to which I also added fresh ginger and reishi mushroom and garlic). Overnight the symptoms progressed to my lungs...a deep cough signifying bronchitis. I had more coconut oil, probably 3 or 4 tablespoons.

Usually when my body is successfully fighting an illness like this, the symptoms gradually subside over a couple of days at best. But in this case, by nightfall of New Years day, ALL my symptoms were absolutely GONE! Wow. I could only imagine those free fatty acids busting up all the influenza viruses one by one as the reason. I have never experienced such a quick and complete turnaround.
Melissa E

The other day my husband came home from work with the flu. He said everyone around him was coming down with it. I had him start taking virgin coconut oil. After two days he came home upset. He complained that he was the only person well enough to go to work, so he was having to do everyone else's jobs. He was the only one in his department that wasn't sick. He almost wishes he hadn't taken the oil so that he could stay home as well.
YA

Some other common viral infections that have been successfully treated with coconut oil include herpes, hepatitis, chicken pox, and measles. Coconut oil is often more effective than commercial antiviral medications.

I am a OBGYN working in Malaysia. I am very interested in holistic medicine and using food as medicine. Early this month a friend gave me a copy of Coconut Cures. *I read it and think it is wonderful. Two weeks ago I had a patient who had genital herpes type 2 infection that started as an itch which she scratched with*

35

her left hand. As a result, she had a herpes infection on her fingers and the skin of the finger tips were peeling, became very painful, and tender, so much so she dare not touch anything with the affected fingers. I treated her with systemic and local Zovirax. The lesion on the fingers did not get better. Then I asked her to apply virgin coconut oil to her fingers. There was marked improvement the next day and soon the pain and peeling were gone.

Dr. Z. Poey

I read in Bruce Fife's book that coconut oil works against lipid coated viruses such as the herpes simplex 1 virus (the virus that causes cold sores). A couple of days ago I got that dreaded tingling in my lips. I was due in the dentist's chair the following day. How embarrassing would it be to have a great big cold sore on my lip!

Not to fear, before going to sleep I smeared some coconut oil on the affected area, and indeed the rest of my lips. It worked a treat. No cold sore! Not even a mark. Unlike Zovirax, which always leaves a visible mark, takes much longer to work, and is far less effective.

GA

I gave someone that I do business with some coconut oil as she has hepatitis C and told me that it has gotten worse and she was so tired all the time. She takes a teaspoon or so a day and told me that her energy has returned and she has more mental clarity. She even looks different, and this has been a transformation in a very short period of time. My niece and my sister are using it for skin issues, one of my friends no longer gets cold sores, and one of my co-workers has eliminated his severe dandruff problem.

JS

I was diagnosed at one time to have "shingles" (the old version of chicken pox) which made my hip's skin feel like it literally was being ironed. My doctor said the only way to deal with it is to take some kind of horribly expensive antibiotic! Since it was still bearable, I did not buy the prescription. I put coconut oil on it

instead, and what do you know. The thing went away in minutes!!!! My sister came to me with the same complaint coming from her doctor (same as mine). I told her to apply coconut oil, and it also worked for her.
MB

Why Use Virgin Coconut Oil?

Since there are many medications available to treat infectious illnesses some people may wonder what need is there for coconut oil? There are several good reasons. You can use coconut oil with other treatments to enhance their effectiveness.

Unlike drugs, coconut oil has no harmful side effects. Drugs, for the most part, are chemicals that are foreign to the human body and, therefore, are inherently toxic to some degree. Even relatively harmless over-the-counter drugs can have undesirable side effects. Not coconut oil. Coconut oil is a food, not a drug. It's a food with healing properties.

One of the drawbacks with using antibiotics is that they tend to kill all the bacteria in the body, including the good bacteria in our intestinal tract. This good bacteria are important because they help to keep the digestive tract functioning properly. Good bacteria produce beneficial nutrients such as vitamin K and some of the B vitamins. They help break down food to release nutrients and prevent the overgrowth of harmful bacteria and yeasts. One of the consequences of frequent antibiotic use is yeast infections. When the good bacteria are killed, yeasts which are not affected by antibiotics, grow unrestrained. They can quickly overrun the intestinal tract causing a yeast infection.

The advantage of using coconut oil is that it does not kill all bacteria. It doesn't harm the good bacteria in the intestinal tract. Plus, it kills Candida, the organism that causes yeast overgrowth. Therefore, using coconut oil can keep the intestinal tract in good shape.

Another important advantage to coconut oil is that it kills viruses. Antiviral drugs may be able to slow viral growth, but they don't kill them. Your immune system must do the fighting. Coconut oil takes an active part along with your immune system in fighting viruses. Currently, it is the only known antiviral substance that can do this.

Coconut oil is often much cheaper than medications and more convenient to use. Coconut oil can be utilized in day to day cooking and food preparation without any added expense. Being a product of nature, rather than a creation from some chemist's laboratory, many people feel safer using it.

While MCFA may be effective in killing many disease-causing microorganisms, they do not kill all of them. In one respect this is good because it doesn't harm friendly gut bacteria. The drawback, however, is that coconut oil will not work against every infection, so you can't rely on it completely for every illness. At times you may need medications or other forms of treatment. So you might want to consult with your health care provider before taking any course of action.

Coconut oil can be helpful, whether it has a direct effect on a particular organism or not, because it tends to strengthen the immune system and make it more effective. In this respect it can be useful to some degree for any type of infection.

How Much Coconut Oil Do You Need?

How much coconut oil is needed to gain protection from infectious disease? There is no hard and fast rule. But if we use mother's milk as a basis for comparison we can get a good approximation. The amount of MCFA a baby receives in mother's milk is known to be effective in preventing illness. If you extrapolate that amount to an average size adult weighing about 150 pounds (75 kg), you would need to consume 3.5 tablespoons (49 grams) of coconut oil a day to get the same protection an infant gets consuming only breast milk.

If you weigh less than 150 pounds you can reduce that. If you weigh more, you can increase it. However, *any* amount is beneficial. Even 1 tablespoon is beneficial. I recommend that for most adults 2-3 tablespoons a day is good as a preventative measure.

If you are struggling with an infectious illness, particularly a serious illness, you may want to increase this amount to 4-6 tablespoons daily. Many doctors have their very sick patients consume this amount.

Coconut oil is not harmful even in very large amounts. I know people who have taken as much as 15 tablespoons a day. But this is only for a few days or weeks at a time. I don't recommend this much on a day-to-day basis. Two to four tablespoons is generally enough for most circumstances.

Although coconut oil is safe, I need to give a word of warning. If you have not been in the habit of eating much oil, if you suddenly start taking 3-4 tablespoons a day you might experience some intestinal discomfort and diarrhea. These symptoms may occur because your digestive system is not accustomed to processing that much oil. Your body needs time to adapt. I suggest that you start off with no more than 1 tablespoon a day and gradually build up. For some people even 1 tablespoon is too much. In that case, drop back to 1 teaspoon and work from there. Three teaspoons equals 1 tablespoon. It may take several months before you feel comfortable with 2-4 tablespoons daily.

Chapter 4

A Super Food

Nature's Perfect Food

As you recall from the previous chapter MCFA are normally attached in groups of three to form medium-chain triglycerides (MCT). Coconut oil is the richest natural source of MCT. Another good source is human breast milk. MCT are a very important component of breast milk. In fact, they are *essential* for the growth, development, and survival of newborn babies.

The antibacterial, antiviral, antifungal, and antiparasitic properties of the medium-chain fatty acids protects newborn infants from infections for the first few months of their lives while they are nursing. MCT not only protect babies from infectious diseases but also protect them from nutritional diseases and promotes proper growth and development. MCT digest very easily and provide a quick and easy source of nutrition thus improving digestion and nutrient absorption.

Unlike the long-chain triglycerides found in most oils, MCT do not need pancreatic digesting enzymes or bile for digestion. Because they digest so quickly, they provide a quick source of nutrition without taxing the enzyme systems of the body. They not only improve the absorption of fats, but enhance the absorption of vitamins and minerals. Therefore, when MCT are present in food, they increase the amount of nutrients that are effectively absorbed into the body. Studies have shown that when premature infants are given formula containing MCT they grow faster and have a higher survival rate. For this reason, coconut oil or

MCT are almost always added to commercial and hospital baby formulas.

For years scientists have recognized the superiority of mother's milk over manmade infant formulas. Formula manufacturers have attempted to imitate the nutritional profile of human milk as closely as possible. Adding coconut oil or MCT makes the formula more like mother's milk.

Mother's milk is nature's perfect food. As hard as scientists try to create the perfect baby formula they can never improve on nature. MCT are in mother's milk to protect infants from infectious disease, aid in digestion, and enhance nutrient absorption which facilitates proper growth and development and improves a baby's chances for survival.

By the way, MCT are saturated fats. They are the same type of saturated fats found in coconut oil. Now some people think all saturated fats are harmful and promote heart disease. This is not true. As you have seen in Chapter 2, coconut oil rich in MCT do not promote heart disease. If MCT don't cause heart disease in nursing infants, some of which nurse up to three years or more, why would they cause heart disease in us? It's hard to imagine nature's perfect food being harmful in any way, especially to newborn infants. Simple logic dictates that MCT, although saturated, do not promote heart disease.

Once a baby is weaned it no longer enjoys the many advantages offered by MCT in mother's milk. However, there is no reason why we cannot continue to take advantage of MCT. Even as adults MCT can provide us with protection against infections and improved digestion and nutrient absorption. This is exactly what medical research has been discovering. For this reason, MCT or coconut oil is being recommended for a variety of digestive and metabolic health concerns.

Improved Digestion

Many people have a difficult time digesting fats. When they eat foods high in fat it gives them indigestion or causes intestinal discomfort. However, since coconut oil digests much easier than other fats many people who have problems with fats can tolerate coconut oil. For people with serious digestive problems coconut oil is the only oil they can use for cooking.

Fried foods make me sick, since they are too hard on my liver. After reading about coconut oil I decided to try frying food at home in coconut oil and find that I can tolerate it fine.
ML

One of the side effects of gastric bypass surgery, where the stomach is shortened as a means to aid in weight loss, is the inability to properly digest fats. Coconut oil is the only oil many of these people can tolerate.

Ever since my gastric bypass eating oils have upset my stomach. Virgin coconut oil never, ever gives me problems.
RI

I had gastric bypass three years ago. Oils and sugars are a big no no. Virgin coconut oil gives me no problems, I can eat it by the tablespoonful and do.
RB

Perhaps the number one digestive problem that people complain of is heartburn or acid reflux. Too many fats can be difficult to digest and may promote acid indigestion. Coconut oil can help relieve it.

After having 25 plus years of severe acid reflux—using the strongest medication barely helped. After one day of using virgin coconut oil I noticed an improvement. By the end of the week it was completely gone and has stopped years of suffering. I've noticed more energy and the loss of junk food cravings. My skin has improved and I can go out in the sun again—no longer a mole hiding in the shade or behind sunscreen. Your book is right—this is nothing short of a "miracle." Praise the Lord.
Sylvia F

Virgin coconut oil cures not just ulcers but also hyperacidity. I had both before I began taking virgin coconut oil regularly. I had been suffering from both for 25 years. My ulcers would occasionally bleed. Both ailments prevented me from enjoying my meals since I had to limit food intake to prevent a bloated feeling

and avoid pains from my ulcers. I also controlled drinking alcoholic and carbonated drinks. With my regular intake of virgin coconut oil I have gotten rid of the pains from both ulcers and hyperacidity. I have developed a very good appetite and can eat and drink anything I want.
Gerry

MCT are metabolized differently from other fats in the body and help to balance blood sugar and reduce sugar cravings.

Since I've taken virgin coconut oil two months ago I'm now migraine free. My hypoglycemia has also been relieved. I just finished reading your book, Coconut Cures. *I'm happy to know from the studies you cited that my body is so amply protected by virgin coconut oil.*
Jim A

After about a week taking the coconut oil my sugar cravings went way down. I used to make 1 gallon of tea with 1 cup sugar, now I make decaf tea with ½ cup sugar and I don't get the munchies much.
RB

The first thing I noticed after three days was that I didn't crave sugar or carbs as much. This was a big thing for me as it was almost an addiction. Now I can take them or leave them. This is so good as it took incredible amounts of willpower to stop me buying chocolate when I went shopping for food.
Kevin

Increased Energy

One of the big differences between LCT and MCT is the way they are metabolized by the body. Among other things, LCT are stored in the body as body fat. MCT, in contrast, are burned to produce energy, and little if any is stored. Because MCT are preferentially used by the body as an immediate source of energy, eating coconut oil produces a boost in energy levels. For most people an increase in energy is most welcome. For some people who have problems with low energy such as those with hypothyroidism or chronic fatigue it can be a blessing.

About two months ago we were led into the knowledge of the wonderful benefits of coconut oil. We dived right in and within 2-3 days of taking coconut oil (3-4 tablespoons daily) I noticed a wonderful difference! I think the best way to describe it is that my physical body felt "happy" and "at peace"! In addition, my energy surge was significant and has continued. My husband gradually began taking it and increasing his dose and now he, too, has had an improvement in his energy level. Previous to consuming coconut oil we often made the comment that we were feeling we had to take a whip to our backs to do what we had to do for the day. We just realized that we have not thought of saying that since beginning the coconut oil regime! We are deeply grateful for this blessing.
Kay K

I started taking coconut oil after I read your book about a month ago. I can't believe what a big difference it has made in my appetite and energy. I usually walk about 45 minutes a day and am usually starved by the time I get done exercising. Now I can walk twice as long and still have energy and not be hungry. I have lost a couple of pounds and feel great. I am 58 years young and wish I would have had this information on coconut oil years ago.
SM

As an (aging) serious competitive athlete (36 year old cyclist/ weight lifter) I feel that, in whatever way, the coconut oil is working in my body it is in some way allowing me to have remarkable recovery from my workouts (I take no other supplementation other than fish oil caps). I have been working out literally 2/3 less then I used to and, for whatever reason, I am getting incredible results from the little bit of time I do put in and feel as if I am as strong, if not stronger than I was in my 20's. It is amazing because as a cyclist they typically peak (and thus retire) at around 30-32 years of age and I don't know where the recovery/strength is coming

44

from other than to say it must in some way be related to the coconut oil!
RO

Coconut oil can be consumed most any time of the day. However, I don't recommend eating it too late at night or before going to bed, as the following example explains.

I noticed that when I took the oil before my bedtime the first week I couldn't fall asleep. All of a sudden I was wide awake. So, I guess it was revving up my metabolism. I stopped taking it at bedtime and fell asleep easily again.
LM

Many people have found it difficult to fall asleep after eating coconut oil late at night. I recommend that people don't eat the oil any sooner than three hours before going to bed. While it can keep you from sleeping at night, it can also help to keep you awake if you need to. Instead of drinking a cup of coffee, a tablespoon of coconut oil can do the trick. Although coconut oil isn't as potent as coffee, its effects tend to last a little longer.

Weight Loss

A health problem that is gaining international attention is the increasing number of people who are overweight and obese. Although we are reducing calories and cutting out fats we are getting fatter. Weight loss diets don't seem to be effective. Even those that seem to work aren't really all that effective because once a person gets off the diet the weight comes right back. The only sure method to keep weight off is to remain on the diet indefinitely. Most diets, however, are so restrictive that no one would want to stick with them permanently. Even two or three months is a chore for most of us.

The best diets are those that can be incorporated into a person's lifestyle without causing major changes. In this way, the diet is more likely to be accepted and maintained. Simply changing the type of fat you eat can have a dramatic impact on your health and on your weight.

One of the effects often reported by coconut oil users is that when they switch to coconut oil they tend to lose excess weight. Even just adding coconut oil into their diet can result in weight loss.

People ask, "How can eating fat help with weight loss?" Coconut oil can help promote weight loss in overweight individuals in several ways. As we learned earlier, coconut oil can help balance blood sugar which tempers sugar and food cravings. If you don't have food cravings you are less likely to snack on cookies, chips, and other weight promoting goodies. We also learned that coconut oil stimulates metabolism and boosts energy levels allowing a person to become more physically active. This causes more calories to be burned. So you tend to snack less and use up more calories by increasing your level of physical activity.

Coconut oil also tends to reduce hunger. When coconut oil is added to a meal you become satisfied sooner and, therefore, eat less. Coconut oil also slows down the digestion so that foods digest more completely. As digestion is slowed, hunger is delayed. Consequently, there is less of a tendency to snack between meals. The overall effect is a reduction in calorie consumption. You eat fewer calories so that there are fewer calories to be converted into body fat. Depending on other aspects of your diet you can experience a significant loss of excess weight as the following people can testify.

I lost 20 pounds when I started using coconut oil—after trying for years to lose weight. I know it was the oil because during the same period my daughter also lost weight, about 10 pounds, just because I had replaced all oils with coconut.

The weight stayed off for a long time, however, I began to be lax in my eating habits and began eating too much of stuff I knew would make me gain weight—empty carbohydrates, it is sometimes hard to do without them in a society that thrives on such stuff! I regained about 7 pounds; but about 2 weeks ago I took myself in hand and am again losing weight, quite rapidly too. I notice that my energy really increased with coconut oil. I can't live without it!
Sharon M

I tried to put on a dress this morning everything I tried was too big or sadly still too small, finally found a 16 dress that was a

bit tight but after being a 20/22 for so long I was sooo pleased to be a 16 again, even if it's a tight 16. I have really been trying to lose weight this year and coconut oil is definitely helping me...I have lost 22 pounds on adding coconut oil to my diet.
ST

The Atkins plan has become a permanent lifestyle for me. I added virgin coconut oil nine months ago. I'm down 55 pounds and my doctor is very happy with my lipid levels.
Anne

I lost nearly 90 pounds in three years using coconut oil. I ate approximately 2500 calorie daily diet with minimal exercises. Of course one needs to eat healthy calories. Adding coconut oil onto a junk food diet probably won't do much good.
AG

Coconut oil not only helps with weight loss but improves overall health. The other benefits you experience may be more important than the weight loss.

I simply take 1 tablespoon three times daily with meals. About three days into this routine I had an energy rush on a Saturday morning that kept me going until well after lunch. I felt like I was about to jump out of my skin and I can't believe how much I got done that day. My mental state of mind seemed to be much sharper, I was able to focus on the tasks at hand without getting sidetracked and I was not exhausted at the end of running my errands, which included traipsing around a huge mall. And it seemed like I was practically running, rather than leisurely walking through the mall as was formerly my habit.

In addition to my energy level, my mood has also been very stable—no up and down swings—even with the onset of PMS! My husband commented yesterday on how soft and silky my skin felt and I have not used any lotion since I started the oil! I'll spare the details on this next particular side effect, but it seems to have given my libido a jump start as well. I guess energy is energy, right?

I have lost two pounds. Taking the oil with my meals seems to give me the "full" feeling a lot faster and my sweet tooth has practically vanished (this from someone who should have bought stock in Hershey long ago!) Ironically, facilitating weight loss was my main reason for trying virgin coconut oil, but with the other wonderful benefits I am experiencing the weight loss aspect almost seems like an afterthought at this point.
Teresa

How much coconut oil do you need to take daily in order to lose weight? The general recommendation is between 2-4 tablespoons daily preferably taken with or before meals. Some people have had good results with just 2 tablespoons or less, while others prefer 4.

As long as I have my 3+ tablespoons of coconut oil in the morning I'm set for the rest of the day. When I have lunch and dinner I don't feel the need to "pig out" as I do at times. I really feel the need for less food.
Dawn

I have been taking approximately 1 teaspoon of virgin coconut oil since June. That one teaspoon, along with keeping an eye on what and how much I eat has resulted in a 20 pound weight loss for me.
Debra

Your book, The Coconut Oil Miracle, *has influenced my family and me immensely. I went from a size 16 to a size 12 in less than a month, just by eating 3 tablespoons of organic coconut oil a day plus by preparing all of my meals with only coconut oil and coconut milk. Our son has just graduated from Chiropractic school in California and from his nutrition seminars and classes he taught us about coconut oil being a healthy fat. Then we found your book and now we won't use any other oil.*
June L

I am 37, obese and have had difficulty losing weight. Using approximately 2 tablespoons of virgin coconut oil daily without intentional dieting or any changes in exercise I lost 14 pounds in five weeks. I ran out of my virgin coconut oil and for the next 4 weeks I maintained my 14 pound loss. I've now used the virgin coconut oil for three weeks again with no other changes in diet or exercise and have dropped 5 pounds. I am very excited about my loss.
Dana B

Some people eat 4 or more tablespoons of coconut oil daily. This is generally more than I recommend, but for some people it works, especially if they are physically active.

I've been using virgin coconut oil for about five weeks—4 or 5 tablespoons per day. I add it to salads (along with virgin olive oil), put a tablespoon in my oatmeal every morning, add it to my pasta sauce, add it to rice, and use it in smoothies.

I've been a competitive athlete for over 25 years, so notice physical changes pretty well right away. I've always competed at a weight of 150 pounds (give or take a pound) and up until I started with virgin coconut oil, that's about my lightest weight I can ever remember (I'm a 56 year old male).

This morning my weight was 140 pounds. It's been pretty amazing to watch my weight fall steadily for the past five weeks. I can never remember being this light.
NV

If you are not accustomed to eating a lot of fat I don't recommend that you start out consuming 3 or 4 tablespoons of coconut oil. Some people can do this, but most can't.

I have just started taking virgin coconut oil two weeks ago and I have noticed several things.

1) My appetite has decreased quite a bit. I don't crave sweets as much, except for certain times of the month.

2) I started out taking about 2-3 tablespoons of virgin coconut oil in the morning, but cut back because it was causing loose stools. I now take about 1 tablespoon.

3) I climb a lot of stairs where I work and used to get very winded, but not very much anymore.

Chris

Oil, any oil, can have a laxative-like effect. Limit yourself to 1 tablespoon at first. The body needs a few weeks to adjust to a higher fat intake. As your body adapts, gradually increase the amount of oil you eat. Highly sensitive people may not even be able to handle 1 tablespoon. In that case start off with 1 teaspoon.

I also recommend that you do not eat the oil all at once, divide it into two or three servings and eat them throughout the day. If you eat 3 tablespoons of coconut oil daily, divide it into three 1 tablespoon servings taken at each meal. If you are only eating 1 tablespoon then divide it into 3 teaspoon sized servings.

Don't just add coconut oil into your diet. For best results in losing weight you need to replace all the other oils you are using with coconut oil. You also need to eat a healthy diet with ample fresh fruits, vegetables, and whole grains. You can't eat cakes and candies every day and expect to magically lose weight. You need to eat sensibly and watch how much you eat.

Some people complain that when they add coconut oil into their diets they don't see the weight loss that others report. A few even report that they gain weight. If this happens to you, look at the types and the amount of food you are eating.

When I finally started looking at what I was eating I was eating way too much. I cut back, continued on with my coconut oil and I am 3 sizes smaller in my jeans and have more energy than ever. I don't weigh myself anymore because the fluctuations can be harmful to one's motivation, or at least some of us. Use a measuring tape or your clothes for a better gauge of what is happening with your body. Put the scale away for awhile.

JS

50

What's the best way to eat coconut oil? Many people eat it by the spoonful just like a dietary supplement. A good quality virgin coconut oil has a light coconut flavor and is very tasty. Some people just can't stand putting oil into their mouths. That's OK. I recommend that you eat the oil with food. Prepare your meals using coconut oil. Cook and bake with it just as you do with other oils.

My daily consumption is 4 tablespoons and I use it a thousand different ways. My breakfast this morning was 2 tablespoons in my pinto beans and rice dish. For dinner I'll use the other 2 tablespoons on my salad. It helps me get warm and I've lost 10 pounds since I started using it a couple of months ago!
Linda

Some people report losing weight simply by adding coconut oil into their diets. But for best results you need to remove all other oils and follow a sensible eating plan.

I am on week 3 of Phase 1 of "The Health Lifestyle Plan" in Dr. Fife's book Eat Fat, Look Thin. *I am following it precisely and am taking 1 tablespoon of coconut oil with each meal. On the first week I lost 8 pounds!*
Sharon G

For those people who are seriously interested in losing weight and losing it permanently I recommend my book *Eat Fat, Look Thin*. See page 79 for more details. If you've tried losing weight using coconut oil and have had only limited success I recommend this book to help you along.

If coconut oil helps people lose weight, what about those who are too skinny? Will they start losing weight when then eat coconut oil? The answer is "no." Coconut oil has a biodirectional or balancing effect; overweight people tend to lose weight while underweight people tend to gain weight. The more overweight a person is the greater the effect coconut oil has on weight loss. As you approach normal weight for your height and build weight loss declines.

Some people are so conscious about their weight that they tend to overemphasize weight loss and are actually too thin. These types of people may actually gain a little weight bringing them more into balance. So if you're looking for a means to become skinny, this isn't it.

Pregnancy and Nursing

Since coconut oil has a tendency to promote weight loss is it good for expecting and nursing mothers? Babies need all the nutrition their mothers can provide so mothers need to be careful about their diets. One of the best things you can do for your baby is to consume ample amounts of coconut oil. As mentioned above, coconut oil has a balancing effect on weight, not a harmful one. If your body needs to gain weight it will help. If it needs to lose weight, again it will help.

Coconut oil is ideal for mothers and their babies. One of the amazing things about coconut oil is that it enriches mother's milk with health promoting MCT. A higher percentage of MCT in the milk will improve digestion, nutrient absorption, and protection against infectious organisms. Eating 2-4 tablespoons a day is one of the best things a nursing mother can do for her child. The child will eat better, sleep better, and feel better. Common health problems such as colic and thrush are dramatically reduced. Mothers often report how their baby's health or growth rate improves with the addition of coconut oil, fed either to the nursing mother or to the baby.

A few months ago I recommended virgin coconut oil to a young mother who was still nursing at the time. This will of course increase the [MCT] content of the mother's milk. The baby became so fond of the milk that she almost choked and could not get enough and she grew 5 centimeters (2 inches) in two weeks when the virgin coconut oil supplementation (of the mother) was started.

At present, the young lady no longer nurses, but she adds one teaspoon of virgin coconut oil to the glass jars which she feeds with a spoon.
HR

I have personal experience with this! In fact, this is why I started taking virgin coconut oil in the first place. My baby was very low weight and I just knew that something wasn't right. Our pediatrician was no help, he said because she hadn't lost weight she was fine. I finally went to a naturopathic doctor and explained my situation (besides the baby gaining only a few ounces, I had postpartum depression). My baby was nine pounds and I'd nursed the last six months. He said that I probably didn't have enough good fats in my system. That would account for my milk not being rich enough in fat to help her grow and it also probably had a great deal to do with my hormones being out of whack and me struggling with postpartum depression. I started taking virgin coconut oil when the baby was five months old. By the time she was seven months old she'd gained three whole pounds! My postpartum depression had disappeared also.

We went back for a weight check when the baby was nine months old and she had gained another two pounds and was not only back on the weight chart, but on the correct curve for her age, etc. I had also noticed that she was developing new skills all at once, that maybe she'd not been able to before. My pediatrician was so impressed he asked me what I'd done. I was a little nervous about telling him, but truthfully, the only thing I'd done differently was to take the virgin coconut oil! So I told him and he never rolled his eyes or treated me like I'd lost my mind. He even wrote it in his chart.

Jan

Not only does the baby receive better nutrition but so does the mother. Even before delivery while the fetus is still developing, MCT aid in its development and protection.

In many Southeast Asian and the Pacific island communities it is a tradition for pregnant women to incorporate coconut oil or coconut into their diets, especially during the last few months before delivery. It is their belief that coconut helps to make deliveries easier and the babies stronger and healthier. Over generations of time they have witnessed how coconut oil protects both the mother and developing child.

I recently received a letter from a person whose friend's baby was literally saved with the use of coconut oil. I'll let her tell the story.

I have something to share with you about virgin coconut oil. My sister in faith (we both belong to the Church of Christ) Mechelle Mandal Tirol, 33 years of age, who at seven months pregnant had a problem with her pregnancy. She underwent an ultrasound to know the gender of her baby. She was shocked to learn that her amniotic fluid had decreased to 9.8 cm. The normal count should be 10 cm or more. She was advised to have another ultrasound a week later. By this time it had decreased to 8.6 cm. She was admitted to the hospital. She was given medications and advised to drink lots of water. After three days in the hospital her AFI (Amniotic Fluid Index) decreased to 6.2 cm.

Her doctor told her that if she reaches the critical level of 4.0 cm, she would have to deliver the baby immediately by Caesarian section. Mechelle was extremely worried because her baby was two months pre-mature.

In addition, she was experiencing some other problems. Fetal movement had dramatically slowed down, she had a urinary tract infection (UTI), and her lips were cracked and very dry.

She convinced her doctor to let her go home so that she could attend church the following day, Sunday, and to ask her minister to pray for her and her unborn child. Another thing, she really wanted to see me and asked my advice regarding virgin coconut oil. Her doctor was very worried with her condition and was very hesitant to let her go home. She made her promise to return on Monday and have another ultrasound. If the result was still negative, for sure she would have the operation.

Sunday afternoon right after church service, she consulted me about virgin coconut oil and told me about her condition. She asked me these questions: "Can virgin coconut oil help me with my condition? How many tablespoons shall I drink?" I remembered what I read in your book that if ever you're not feeling well, double the dose. I told her to drink 30ml (2 Tbs) right away when she arrived home, another 30ml before bedtime and 30ml the following day after breakfast. Pray hard, be positive and hope for the best. Her ultrasound was scheduled for 10:00 AM the following day.

Monday afternoon she called me and was very ecstatic with the result of the ultrasound. Her AFI had increased from 6.2 cm to 7.3 cm. She felt better now. Her UTI has gone and no more drying of her lips. And that from only 90ml (6 Tbs) of virgin coconut oil. What an amazing miracle!

Five days later her AFI measured 8.0 cm. Fetal movement which had slowed down during this ordeal also improved. The doctors were surprised with the results and kept asking what had she done. Mechelle wouldn't tell them. No caesarian necessary. As of this writing the child and mother are doing well.

I still could hardly believe that the oil can really make a difference, can save people's lives and unburden them with anxieties as to whatever health condition they are in. God is really soooooo good for giving us the coconut—the Tree of Life.

Thank you so much Dr. Bruce for taking time to read my letter.
Rosemarie R.

The coconut palm is aptly titled the "Tree of Life" This is what the Pacific Islanders call it because they know of its many health promoting properties.

Chapter 5

A Multipurpose Health Tonic

Throughout history coconut oil has been used worldwide as both a food and as a medicine. Since the earliest of times it was recognized for its remarkable healing properties. In the Pacific islands coconut oil served as the basis for their medicine. Coconut oil was applied topically, taken internally, and combined with various herbs and plant extracts. In India coconut oil has played an important role for thousands of years in Ayurvedic medicine. In China ancient medical textbooks going back 2,000 years described the use of coconut in treating and curing no less than 69 diseases. When archeologists uncovered King Tutankhamen's tomb in Egypt in the early 1920s they discovered among the relics an ancient medical text dating back to about 1300 B.C. In this book were references to the medicinal use of coconut oil.

Today the use of coconut oil is kept alive in various forms of traditional medicine around the world. In Fiji and other Pacific islands it is used as a topical ointment to heal injuries and rejuvenate skin and muscle. In Central and South America coconut oil is consumed by the cupful to overcome infectious disease. In the Philippines it is used orally and topically for just about every illness imaginable.

In recent years modern medical science has taken an interest in coconut oil. Research has been unlocking the secrets to the healing properties of this remarkable oil. What researchers are learning is truly remarkable.

Published medical studies have documented numerous health benefits associated with coconut oil and medium-chain fatty acids. Studies show that coconut oil improves insulin secretion and utilization of blood glucose; improves vitamin and mineral absorption; supports immune system function; protects against cancer; blocks the harmful effects of many toxins; supports thyroid function; and helps protect against liver, kidney, and gallbladder disease. It is no wonder why coconut oil has been used so extensively throughout history for its healing properties.

Oxidation and Free Radicals

The medium-chain saturated fatty acids in coconut oil are chemically very stable. One of the problems with most other vegetable oils is their lack of stability. Polyunsaturated fats are very delicate and easily damaged by exposure to oxygen, sunlight, and heat. When polyunsaturated oils are exposed to these conditions they begin to oxidize, that is, they start to go rancid. Rancid oils are dangerous.

When oil oxidizes it creates toxic molecules known as free radicals. Free radicals are highly reactive molecules that attack neighboring molecules, causing them to also become free radicals, which in turn, attack other molecules in a continuous destructive chain reaction. Once a molecule has been transformed into a free radical it is permanently damaged. Cells and tissues that contain damaged molecules cannot function properly.

Table 1. Disease and Free Radicals

Some of the most common conditions involving free-radical degeneration:

Heart disease	Asthma	Atherosclerosis	Hay fever
Cancer	Food allergies	Stroke	Prostate hypertrophy
Diabetes	Ulcers	Psoriasis	Cataract
Eczema	Colitis	Acne	Constipation
Arthritis	Chronic fatigue	Lupus	Alzheimer's disease
Varicose veins	PMS	Hemorrhoids	Parkinson's disease
Failing memory	Seizures	Senility	Prostitis
Kidney stones	Phlebitis	Gout	Multiple sclerosis
Depression	Insomnia	Dysmenorrhea	Fibrocystic breast disease

Free-radical damage is linked to the loss of tissue integrity and to physical degeneration. As cells are attacked by free radicals the tissues become progressively impaired. Researchers have identified at least 60 common health problems associated with free radicals (see table 1). Free radicals don't necessarily cause all of these diseases, but they are involved at least as accomplices. In fact, it has been suggested that most of the damage caused by disease is actually the result of the accompanying free-radical destruction and not from the disease process itself.

Infections, injuries, radiation, toxins and pollutants are just a few of the things that can promote free-radical generation. We are exposed to free-radical forming influences all the time. Free radicals are continually in our bodies. Fortunately, we have a natural defense against them in the form of antioxidants. Antioxidants stop free radicals from forming and block free-radical chain reactions. We get antioxidants from the foods we eat. Vitamins A, C, and E function as antioxidants. Minerals such as zinc and selenium are used in the formation of antioxidant enzymes manufactured in our bodies.

Free radicals are continually being formed in our bodies and, consequently, antioxidants are constantly being used up fighting them off. If antioxidant reserves become depleted free radical damage increases. Low antioxidant status can promote or aggravate many of the conditions listed in Table 1.

One of the problems with polyunsaturated and, to a lesser degree, monounsaturated oils is their vulnerability to oxidation inside the body. If antioxidant reserves are low they can generate copious amounts of free radicals. On a cellular level inside the body MCFA from coconut oil can act as antioxidants by protecting polyunsaturated and monounsaturated oils from oxidation. Consuming coconut oil on a regular basis can help protect you from conditions associated with free radicals.

Inflammation

Inflammation is a defense process initiated by the body to bring about healing. When there is an injury or infection, the inflammation response automatically kicks in. When it does, circulation of the blood increases into the infected area. This can cause swelling, generate heat, and increase pain. This process brings in an increased number of white blood cells to fight the infection and speed healing.

When inflammation works the way it is supposed to, it speeds healing. However, if inflammation is constantly being stimulated it can become a problem. Inflammation accompanies many health problems. If the problem continues, inflammation can become chronic causing a great deal of pain and discomfort. Chronic inflammation can damage tissues and promote the growth of scar tissue. Atherosclerosis or hardening of the arteries is a result of chronic inflammation. If the arteries are chronically inflamed scar tissue, fat, and calcium are continually being deposited. This eventually leads to hardening of the arteries and blockage of the artery canal, with the end result being a heart attack or stroke.

Numerous health problems are associated with chronic inflammation. Besides heart disease you have diabetes, arthritis, Crohn's disease, lupus, multiple sclerosis, ulcerative colitis, eczema, psoriasis, and others. Coconut oil users have reported relief from symptoms associated with all of these conditions. One of the reasons coconut oil may be effective is that it soothes the fire of inflammation. The standard medical treatment for inflammation is anti-inflammatory drugs. Although the anti-inflammatory effects of coconut oil are not as strong as those of drugs, unlike drugs it has no undesirable side effects and often brings about permanent healing rather than just reducing inflammation.

Coconut Oil's Multiple Benefits

Coconut oil's ability to improve digestion and nutrient absorption, increase energy, boost the immune system, fight off infections, block the formation of destructive free radicals, and ease chronic inflammation makes it a powerful tool for promoting better health.

No other oil can compare to the health promoting and healing potential associated with coconut oil. For this reason, coconut oil can have a positive effect on a variety of health problems. Because coconut oil seems to work with such a number of health concerns, health practitioners familiar with using coconut oil often recommend its use for just about any and all conditions. Although it may not help with every problem, it certainly will not hurt. Coconut oil is not harmful and may do a lot of good. Even if it doesn't relieve one particular symptom it is still doing good because it has so many other benefits. It may not cure your appendicitis but it will improve digestion, strengthen your immune system, give you more energy, etc. Often people start using the oil for one problem and find it relieves another.

Aches and Pains

One of the comments I often hear from those using coconut oil is that it helps relieve aches and pains associated with a variety of conditions. Arthritis, gout, fibromyalgia, and even miscellaneous undiagnosed pains of unknown origin see improvement as the following testimonies can verify.

I was walking and golfing as my exercise program, on weekends 18 holes and almost every day after work 9 holes at least. My heels started to ache constantly. I had to leave the golf course frequently, and could barely walk from my truck to my house when I got home. I heard about virgin coconut oil (VCO), starting reading about its ability to reduce inflammation, and thought I'm desperate enough to do it, as I was about ready to give up golf.

So I started taking VCO three times a day. The heels of my feet felt better right away, but only by about half. I was happy with that. I never stopped golfing. But my feet continued to get a little better every day, and after a month and a half, I was completely healed. I knew this when I walked 18 holes 5 days in a row. Later at night my feet felt normal with no pain, nor was there any pain the next morning.

As a side bonus, the calluses on the fingers of my left hand were thick and flakey from playing the guitar. I was having to file them down to be able to play, and my finger tips were tender. That all went away. I still have calluses, but they are pliable now, I don't have to file them, and my finger tips are not tender any more. I can play pretty much as long as I want to now.
Rodney L

I started using Virgin Coconut oil just about 3 weeks ago. I had been suffering with arthritis and back problems. I used to have a problem just getting up out of my seat and since I have been using coconut oil I just get right up with no problems. I thought I had to get a new mattress because my back was hurting so bad but now I have no problems (I am still going to get a new mattress anyway). I just want to say that I am sold on this coconut oil and have recommended it to family and friends and they have and they are telling me great results from it.
Annette R

It worked for my gout. I no longer have any type of attacks for over 9 months now...My gout was so bad I would wake up howling in the middle of the night from a dead sleep. I couldn't stand any type of pressure on the foot or feet (depending on the attack). I wore multiple layers of wool socks to add heat to the feet, used heating pads when stationary, and went through countless styles of shoes trying to find comfort. Now I just wear plain old cheap flip-flops on bare feet. Walk all I want and never think about my feet.
RB

I am 68 years old. I have had fibromyalgia for the past 8 years. For the past two months have been taking 3 tablespoons of coconut oil a day. The pain has greatly lessened and I've never slept better than I do now.
Naomi M

For several years I had arthritis. I would get up out of a chair like an 80-year-old lady and walk bent over for 8-10 steps. It was very difficult for me to sit on something hard like the floor and very difficult to get up from the floor. Stairs were taxing and painful.

Five years ago we completely got rid of all the oils we had been using and used completely virgin coconut oil. We tried to achieve the magical amount of 3-4 tablespoons a day but we did not always get that much into our diet. Gradually, over a three

month period of time the pain lessened until one day I woke up and realized the pain was gone. My arthritis (all in my hips) as well as muscle stiffness went away. It has been five years and the arthritis has never returned.
AF

I am a 38 year old who has inherited osteoarthritis and have the knees of someone much older. Both parents have undergone complete knee replacement in both knees, so I figured I didn't stand a chance. The wear in my knees amazed the doctor. I haven't done anything to cause damage to my knowledge, just plain old heredity. Anyway, I started using the virgin coconut oil on the advice of my Mom, and after about two weeks, the swelling I had went down. My knees don't seem to bother me hardly at all any more. I can squat and stretch, plus use the elyptic trainer at the gym with no adverse effects. So, I would definitely attribute this to the use of the virgin coconut oil.
Laurie

Because of a motorcycle accident when I was 22 (now 51), my leg and knee has always been a problem. Especially with age the problem has worsened. Since I work on the computer for hours on end the knee and leg tend to swell and cause lots of pain. Upon getting up and trying to walk after being seated for so long, it is hard to even walk, that is until the virgin coconut oil. For some reason, after taking [coconut oil] for about 5-6 days I noticed when getting up to walk the knee was not swollen as before, and best of all, NO DEBILITATING PAIN!
Laura

The results with coconut oil have been so striking that doctors and nutritionists have taken notice and are recommending it to their patients. Even multiple sclerosis (MS) patients who suffer from a great deal of pain are responding favorably.

We have tried virgin coconut oil with a few MS patients, who are cured after consuming virgin coconut oil for two and a half

months. MS affects brain and nerve tissue and was incurable until now.
Dr. T.C. Cheng

Allergies
Many people report relief from allergy symptoms with the use of coconut oil.

I use coconut oil when my allergy acts up and I start sneezing, but this time I put it in the walls of my nostrils, just before the sensitive parts. It works. I also use it instead of the nasal sprays because of what I've read about those nasty sprays. It works too. Clears the air passage.
MB

I have always been plagued by various skin problems brought about by allergic reactions to a great number of stimulations from dust to almost everything I ate. My reactions would all come out on my skin. Coconut oil managed to cleanse me in and out and has improved my resistance to the things I was previously so allergic to. I have not taken my allergy medicines nor have I taken any shots since I've been drinking the oil. Amazing.
Popi L

We have been using virgin coconut oil for 2 years now and my wife has hardly had hay fever since. Before that she had it all of the time and often had to take antihistamines. She has had only about 2 or 3 since.
Ian G

Hormones
For many people coconut oil has a balancing effect on hormones. Hormone imbalances can affect all aspects of our life including our mood.

63

I have been using coconut oil for about a year now. It is an amazing oil that has made a lot of changes in me. It's wonderful. I am able to lay in the sun (in Florida) and I don't even need to put suntan lotion on and I don't burn or peel or get dry skin. My skin is much better. My hair is much shinier and I have more energy than I ever had before. I also was a very irritable person and using the oil I am calmer and not so ugly.

Carol T

I just wanted to let the guys know that coconut milk has had a wonderful side effect in my 56-year-old husband. He's been taking testosterone shots for a year now with some good, but limited effects. However, after a couple months on the coconut milk instead of being the pursuer, I'm the pursued (big grin).

RI

Prostate problems have been traced back to imbalances in hormone levels. Enlarged prostate is very common in middle aged and older men. This condition causes frequent urination, especially at night.

In the last three and a half months the only change in my diet to amount to anything significant is using coconut oil and taking 6 mg of melatonin before retiring each night. So far the most noticeable effects have been a more deeper sleep and for the last month, I have not had to urinate during the night after I went to bed. I do not even have the feeling I need to when I wake up. I have not experienced this long sought relief in 20 or more years and it is welcome.

Tracy

I'm 62 years old. About two years ago I started experiencing strong, sudden urges to urinate. The urge said "Gotta go, gotta go!" But there wasn't much to come out. I started on coconut oil about two months ago. I eat about 3.5 tablespoons a day. Since then I have noticed an improvement. I'd say that I'm almost back to normal.

DB

Miscellaneous Health Problems

Coconut oil appears to help relieve the symptoms associated with a variety of conditions, including some serious ones such as diabetes and hypothyroidism. Often unexplained conditions are also relieved.

In my clinical practice at St. Luke's Medical Center I use virgin coconut oil for the elderly in relation to physiologic changes that occur with aging. Virgin coconut oil can address sensory losses, tooth and gum problems, changes in the intestinal tract, changes in the immune system, changes in body composition, and changes that come with menopause and andropause...A combination of old age and malnutrition makes older people vulnerable to pneumonia, UTI, and bedsores. Virgin coconut oil can help fight infection in the early stages. Take the case of a 76-year-old who developed painful herpes zoster on his trunk. The antibiotic cream given to him only lasted for one application because the area affected was so wide. But when virgin coconut oil was applied all over the skin for a week, the patient reported relief from itch and the lesions dried up.
Eliza Perez Francisco, MD

I have suffered with systemic Candida for years and in just 3 weeks I've gone through the die-off of the Candida and have NO cravings for sweets, breads, pasta, or any simple carbs. I don't snack and have to remind myself to eat 4-5 small meals a day. I've lost 5 pounds, have good energy and clearer thinking—no more foggy brain!

My husband is an insulin dependent type 2 diabetic. His fasting blood sugar was never under 140 but it has been ranging between 110-120 since eating virgin coconut oil. He also rubs a little on his balding scalp where he had a persistent rash and scaly scalp and just one night we could see the difference. Today his scalp is pink and healthy looking.
BH

February 1 I began taking 3 tablespoons of virgin coconut oil every day. I had had fairly severe symptoms of hypothyroid and

adrenal exhaustion, and these symptoms disappeared within the first week. I immediately began to sleep through the night, wake up alert and refreshed after only eight hours of sleep (unusual for me). I also felt cheerful and energetic.
KH

I used to go through prodigious night sweats when I slept. Sometimes my blankets would be soaking wet in the morning. At other times I would get cold very easily. Since taking lots of coconut oil regularly I have no night sweats and no feeling of alternating between hot and cold.
AG

One of the huge benefits of using coconut is that it can save you money as well as improve your health. Using coconut daily can reduce your dependence on costly medications. Coconut oil being a natural food, rather than a manmade chemical, has no harmful side effects. It is completely safe to use.

It's almost a year since I began taking virgin coconut oil. Since then I have not taken any medicine. My sinusitis is gone, my son's asthma is gone, common colds are no longer common in our household. My wife's arthritic pain is gone...Even my energy (I play tennis) is enhanced. One very noticeable benefit is our bowel movements. We seldom get constipated.
Tony M

I used to have restless leg syndrome and it drove me crazy. What I used to do before I started living healthier is take a lot of Xanax. I also had depression and took antidepressants. At the time I ate a very low fat diet (almost no fat and NO saturated fat). Then I read how your brain is composed of a lot of fat (including saturated fat and cholesterol) and restricting fat can mess up your neurological connections. I started reading about the benefits of coconut oil and other fats I had previously avoided, like butter and the cholesterol in eggs. After I started taking coconut oil and using butter and eggs, I stopped my Xanax and antidepressant

66

(which I had taken for nine years). My depression and restless legs are gone.
Mary H

We have had a very positive experience using virgin coconut oil with our 6-year-old daughter. From around the age of 2 she had a form of undiagnosed arthritis that would make her immobile on many days. The pediatrician put her on Vioxx for awhile (this was before it was banned) which we weren't happy with, but it wasn't much fun seeing her on the worst days crawling like a baby because it hurt too much to walk or lying on her back much of the day because it hurt too much to play. We cut out vegetable oils from our diet 18 months ago and replaced them with virgin coconut oil and butter. Soon after we weaned her off the Vioxx and she has hardly complained of pain since.
Ian G

In 1987 I was diagnosed with what was then called Post Viral Syndrome, now ME/CFS/CFIDS. I'd had a serious bout of flu in 1986 from which I did not recover properly, although my health had been slowly deteriorating since mid 1985. I had a severe relapse in 1993 following a flu vaccination. From this point I was often house and/or bed bound. My husband (my rock) and I have been everywhere and tried everything.

To cut a long story short, it was suggested by a doctor in London that I should see an endocrinologist in Brussels – at that point I was on hydrocortisone (blood pressure down to 80/30 which precipitated the prescription).

The endocrinologist always spent a lot of time lecturing us on diet. Lecturing is not too strong a word, he was very insistent that I should use coconut oil for cooking and not olive oil. Your book, The Coconut Oil Miracle, was shown to us along with a tub of oil. He was against the prevailing low fat dogma, saying that fat is required by the body for making hormones.

The second strand of his diet theory was that I should eat a paleolithic type diet: no grains, sugar, dairy. Not too much fruit, loads of vegetables and salad, plus meat, fish nuts and seeds. My complaint was that I like yoghurt, so I was allowed two a week as a concession. This diet is very healthy especially when combined with the coconut oil and over time I recovered to a point where I decided to get off the meds. Since September 2004 I have been off all meds and my health since then has improved dramatically.

I think that my immune system is getting back to normal as I had flu two months ago, was acutely ill and then recovered normally instead of languishing with fluey symptoms for months as previously. I have a few minor problems left, but I am hopeful that another six months should see me right.

My husband is also very healthy on this diet. He has lost 35 pounds (I lost 7 pounds after dropping the steroids, back to a normal weight of 125 pounds). Eighteen months ago just after turning forty he took up squash again. As one of his friends commented, most people give up squash at 40, not take it up again!

Jo W

Coconut oil has shown to be effective in relieving symptoms associated with a wide variety of health problems. Since it is completely non-toxic and safe it can be used for just about any health problem. It may not ease every condition but since it isn't harmful, remember it's a food and not a drug, it can be used without worry.

Chapter 6

Beautiful Skin and Hair

A Natural Skin Lotion

Virgin coconut oil is absolutely the best natural all purpose skin and hair care product you can use. I have never seen any lotion, cream, or other product work as well as virgin coconut oil for healing and rejuvenating the skin and beautifying the hair. If you have rough, dry, flaky skin virgin coconut oil will make it smooth, soft, and younger looking in no time. I've seen people who have had dry, chapped hands for years develop soft, smooth hands in a matter of days. Coconut oil is good for just about any type of skin condition. It can help eliminate skin and nail fungus, dandruff, psoriasis, warts, moles, and even aging spots. It also speeds healing of injuries such as cuts, burns, and insect bites. It even protects against skin cancer. I have never seen anything work as well as coconut oil.

If you start using coconut oil on your skin be prepared for some changes as noted by the following people.

One of my Tai Chi classmates asked me if I wanted to try a new product that their company was developing. I had been buying essential patchouli oil from her and she wanted to know if I was interested in virgin coconut oil. "What does it do?" I inquired and she said it was very good for the skin. Now for me those were magic words!

I have always been plagued by various skin conditions. It was so bad that my friends, out of pity, would give me the numbers of their dermatologists so I could get help. At that point my bathroom already resembled a small apothecary so I was willing to try anything.

From the first time I oiled myself from head to foot it was immediate love. I guess, even if I had not known it then, the light yummy smelling oil would save me. After a month of religiously using it the compliments started pouring in and they haven't stopped—three years later.

Now when I visit the cosmetologist to get a facial they marvel at how my skin resembles that of a baby. Now that kind of compliment was something I was completely unaccustomed to. And instead of selling me their services, they insist I don't leave without giving them my source for the oil. Even doctors who have treated my numerous skin conditions marvel at how truly healthy my skin looks.

I do not have any visible scars from my war-torn dermal past. Friends who've never seen me before do not believe the stories of scars over scars over scars, while old friends vouch that it's been such a transformation. I'm practically a walking-talking signboard for what this simple, yet wonderful, gift from nature can do, and continues to do.

I'm convinced I shall never be without it and I will continue to tell those who care to listen about how it has changed my life for the better.

Popi L

I have been using coconut oil for about three weeks and have been amazed at the benefits so far. For the first time in my life, my oily skin is actually under control! Who would of ever thought that putting oil on you face before bed would control the oil all day long? I had red, scabby-type rashes on my calves for over 9 months. After one week of coconut oil, they are almost gone. My fingernails are stronger. My heels aren't rough, dry and tearing my hose anymore. My skin is softer and smoother. I love how it absorbs completely into the skin.

Shari

I just wanted to share a compliment my husband gave me a few days ago. Now keep in mind that my husband is not one to just hand out compliments lightly! When he gives a compliment it is a total miracle in my estimation, so that is why I am here to tell you about my ecstatic overjoy when he told me my skin sure was looking soft and smooth lately! Trying not to act too excited and holding my composure, I told him it must be the coconut oil. Yeahhh!
Mary

Coconut oil can work wonders as a topical skin cream, but it can also beautify your skin from the inside out. Eating the oil affects the health of your skin. This makes sense because when you eat the oil it affects the entire body and improves skin health from the inside out.

Since I started using coconut oil for frying, don't do much frying, baking occasionally and one to three tablespoons daily, the skin on my elbows and knees changed from dry to smooth. And a couple of months into the coconut oil use part of my black spot came up to the skin surface and I brushed it away. Today several months later the rest of my black spot was on the surface and I just brushed it off. Now there is no black spot. Now it is gone. A light pink spot appears to be on the surface. I had the black spot for some 15 years about a half inch above my right eyebrow, it was about 1/8-inch in diameter and well below the surface of the skin but quite visible.
LO

Beautify Your Hands and Feet
The hands and feet are probably the most abused parts of our bodies. They are generally the first to show signs of wear and tear. If you want something to improve the texture and appearance of your hands and feet virgin coconut oil (VCO) is the answer.

I have not been on virgin coconut oil for long but I can tell you what it has done for me so far. I have been putting it on my cracked and often times bleeding heels that somewhat resemble cement. After using the oil on my heels for five nights the cracks have completely healed and my feet are softer than they have been in years. I have also been using it on my body and on my face as a moisturizer and two small burned spots on my face have completely gone away.

Diana

I have become such a missionary for coconut that my family and friends have begun to call me "Coconut" or simply "Nut" for short! But even the skeptics are impressed with the results they are getting. I had cracked, dry, smelly feet that no amount of salve and lotions helped. In two days the feet were soft and non-smelly, and the fungus much improved. My skin needed help and it is very much improved, especially my hands. They look 20 years younger.

Marilyn R

My right thumb has eczema that comes and goes depending on my immune system performance. My dermatologist prescribed a very expensive steroid cream to treat it when it's active. Three weeks ago, the eczema was making my thumb "weep," itchy, and red. Instead of putting on the steroid cream, I applied VCO and covered it with gauze. The following morning the redness was gone and the skin became dry. I continued to apply VCO three times a day and after a few days the thick flaky dead skin was gone and my thumb is smooth again. Another bonus is a smoother complexion as I use VCO as a "night cream." Since then I have replaced my cooking oil with VCO and my children are getting used to it. Thank God for VCO!

Lorna P

My 92-year-old mom has nerve damage in her feet and uses coconut oil to massage her feet and ankles. Lo and behold all that nasty purple bruised looking effect on her ankles and feet is gone after six months of greasing up nightly with coconut oil. This stuff is impressive.

NS

72

The first thing I noticed is how it has improved my 74-year-old hands that were in deplorable condition. My hands are now very smooth, hangnails disappeared in two days, age spots are fading out, the veins are less prominent. Blood pressure, which was slightly elevated, has gone down about 20 points. I appear to have more stamina and feel more energetic, but that might be because I think I should. My skin looks a whole lot better overall—maybe the wrinkles will all disappear! My daughter had terrible feet—cracked and rough and smelly, and no amount of lotions and treatments helped much. It only took about three days for them to get soft and smooth, and the smell is gone.
MA

Face and Complexion

Some people have been hesitant to put coconut oil on their faces because they feel their skin is too oily and adding more oil will compound the problem. They also fear that it may increase the appearance of acne. However, coconut oil improves the complexion and helps prevent acne.

I use virgin coconut oil on my face every evening before I go to bed. I clean my face, dry it, then apply virgin coconut oil—not too much, very lightly. When I wake up in the morning my acne is dried up and looks 100% better with each application I make. I find that if I use it before I go to bed it works much better than when I use it in the morning when my pores are opened and exposed to the environment. Seems to work for me!
Terri M

My face broke out for almost 4 months and I sometimes had these huge breakouts that would go away sometimes as quickly as they came on. When I would get one that was weeping I would make a paste of coconut oil and coconut flour and it would soak it right up. I no longer have breakouts.
JS

I started putting virgin coconut oil on my face yesterday and wow my skin is smooth and soft as a baby's bum. At first if felt really greasy but my skin soaked it all up within 15 minutes. No greasy residue at all.

FI

My son washes his face at least two times a day and puts on the virgin coconut oil. It's working great! I'm so glad I found this before my little girl (now 13) has a problem with acne. We can keep her face clear before it ever starts! I have also noticed that the brown spots on the tops of my hands are peeling off, slowly but surely the age spots are disappearing.

Robin

I am 25 years old. I just started using virgin coconut oil 3 weeks ago. I have very sensitive skin, skin redness, pimples in my back and chest and big pores.

Since I was 16 years old I always bought different kinds of expensive cosmetics, creams and facial mask to avoid and to get rid of my pimples. These products caused me only more blemishes and my face turned dry. I noticed if my skin gets dried from different kinds of cosmetics and creams and facial mask I only get more blemishes. I had back pain last month since I am working in the office 9 hours a day. My cousin massaged my back with the virgin coconut oil and the next day I noticed that my pimples on my back went dry and it feels so smooth. So I started applying it on my face daily and all over the body. And now I have a very smooth face and it has its moisture again. My skin redness, pimples, big pores are all gone. It really helps a lot and I can really recommend the virgin coconut oil.

Jen

Many people have reported how coconut oil applied to the face and body daily prevents acne. In some cases, however, when a person first starts to use the oil acne may temporarily increase. The oil in this case is acting as a cleanser or detoxifier and pulling toxins out of the skin. Acne may increase for a few weeks but as the skin expels the toxins the complexion improves.

Dermatitis

Dermatitis is characterized by inflammation of the skin. Rashes, hives, psoriasis, eczema, and even fungal infections can be involved in the occurrence of dermatitis. Coconut oil can often help relieve much of the inflammation, pain, and itching associated with dermatitis.

I had a skin rash that did not go away on my arms and the back of my thighs. Well I have used coconut oil for two weeks and it's all gone. After everything I had tried, something so simple, cheap, and so easy to use worked better than anything.
Diane

I have very bad eczema on my hands and arms and have tried every prescription cream. The only thing that has worked in the past is a large injection of cortisone, which greatly lowers your immune function. I happened to buy some coconut oil for my daughter's thick and curly hair, hoping it would moisturize it. By chance I put some on my eczema and it really helped. So I tried an experiment, I stopped using the non-steroidal cream and just put on the coconut oil. I was amazed that my eczema felt so much better and is starting to go away after only a week. For the first time all winter I don't have any open skin cracks on my hands (very painful!) and my skin is healing.
Jen C

Throughout most of my childhood and into adulthood I had severe eczema covering most of my body and my doctor at the University of Michigan told me to use only coconut oil and cocoa butter on my hair and skin. It has worked for me for decades now.
MJH

Two relatives of mine, both avid golfers, have very itchy thick hives on their backs. They have been to good dermatologists and

75

were given prescription creams that cost too much and yet their hives did not go away. They asked for my cream, and overnight the thick hard hives have softened, and after a few days the hives disappeared with no trace.

It has also been used by one of them for an infected big toe. The infection cleared in a matter of three days.
   MB

I've been applying it to a rash that I have on my leg. A rash that my doctors have no idea what it is. First a doctor said it was a heat rash then some sort of inflectional rash (whatever that means) and on and on. Nothing they gave me made it go away. Since putting the virgin coconut oil on it is almost completely gone and I believe will be completely gone in another day or so.

I have also been applying it to the heels of my feet that have always been so rough and lately have been cracking and bleeding. For the past week I've been putting the virgin coconut oil on them twice a day. Today I noticed they are much softer and have not cracked and bled at all for days.
   Ruth

Doctors interested in natural approaches to patient care who are actively using virgin coconut oil are reporting positive results.

Based on my clinical practice at Makati Medical Center, nutritional supplements of virgin coconut oil lower the severity of psoriasis secondary infection and atopic dermatitis cases.
   Vermen Verallo-Rowell, MD
   Dermatologist

As seen in the above cases virgin coconut oil can work wonders in relieving many types of dermatitis. Since dermatitis can have any number of causes, the response each person will experience may vary. If the cause of the dermatitis is localized in the affected skin, virgin coconut oil is very effective as a treatment. Dermatitis can also be a symptom of a problem in another part of the body such as the liver or colon. Toxins draining from these organs may be expelled though the

76

skin causing the dermatitis. In this case, applying virgin coconut oil on the affected skin may only bring mild, temporary relief. The following is an excellent example of this.

For nearly eight months my former father-in-law was suffering from unexplained rashes all over his body. He went to the dermatologist and his regular general practitioner, etc. He was prescribed antibiotics, topical medications, you name it. Nothing seemed to help. When one area was treated, the rash migrated to another part of his body. Finally, during a routine dental exam the dentist discovered a "silent" abscess. It had not been painful because the infection had been draining into his system. Within days after the abscess was treated the rashes disappeared.

If after using coconut oil the skin doesn't show significant improvement, the problem is likely caused by a condition somewhere else in the body. In this case another approach needs to be taken.

Hair and Scalp

Coconut oil helps bring out the natural color in hair, give it a healthy shine, and protect it from damage. The oil also works on the scalp to improve skin health and get rid of dandruff.

A good procedure to follow is to massage a liberal amount of coconut oil into the hair and scalp. Wait about 15-30 minutes for the oil to soak in then wash it out with shampoo. The hair and scalp will look and feel fantastic. After washing, some people like to rub a small amount of oil between their hands and brush it through their hair. This final step gives the hair added shine and keeps it from tangling or becoming frizzy.

I used to have very dry scalp. I color my hair and that was my problem. My ears were even dry. I started melting virgin coconut oil, applying it all over my hair and scalp, then put a vinyl shower cap on and apply warm heat from my hair dryer for a few minutes. I would keep the cap on for awhile afterwards to let the oil soak in. I only needed to do this three times. I would put the oil on the outer edges of my ears and put the cap over them too. I did this twice a week. Now once a week, I rub oil into my scalp a few minutes before my shower (if I have time I'll wait an hour). My hair looks and feels better and my scalp and ears are not dry. My hair used to fall out terribly and that has stopped.

TB

Since reading your book The Coconut Oil Miracle *three months ago I have been ingesting at least three tablespoons of coconut oil daily. I love its taste. After showering I massage virgin coconut oil over my entire body. Before washing my hair, I massage generous amounts of coconut oil into my scalp, then I read for an hour or so before washing my hair. Wow! What used to feel like straw now feels like silk, even my barber asked what was I doing to make it so soft and shiny. Naturally, I told him about coconut oil.*

RM

I do a "hair treatment." I massage warmed virgin coconut oil into my hair and scalp. Then I put on a shower cap for 20 minutes or so. This got rid of my flaky, itchy and dry scalp. I then wash my hair with a bar shampoo and condition lightly. Hardly any tangles. After I have combed out my hair I then apply a few drops of virgin coconut oil to the ends of my hair. My hair never feels oil or greasy, it absorbs the virgin coconut oil nicely. Just looks healthy and shiny.

Lizmarie

I find that applying a small amount of virgin coconut oil (about a spot in my palm the size of a quarter) and massage in thoroughly then blow dry and forget about frizzy hair and split ends. Neat!

BB

It made my hair so soft and gave it moisture again...I don't like to judge things too quickly, but I honestly could not believe just one application did such wonders! I would imagine different people will have different results, but I'm sure you can't go wrong. So far, since the one treatment I am not flaking as much as I had.

78

It feels good to run my fingers through my hair and feel the silk like texture which I have not had in a long time.
    Tonia

My hair, when freshly washed and dried can be a bit flyaway so yesterday I tried using virgin coconut oil as a pomade of sorts. Put a tiny bit in my palm, rubbed my hands together till most of it was absorbed, then rubbed them over my hair. It was lighter and worked better than the expensive stuff my hair stylist sold me!
    Julia

I have been using the oil for about two weeks. My skin looks great, no more dryness. I used to have very dry skin. My hair looks great, soft and shiny, no more frizz. And my scalp is no longer dry. Also, my eyelashes have grown longer and thicker! This is a plus I did not expect. I now make an effort to apply a bit of oil with a clean mascara brush each morning/night.
    LM

Some people report that regular coconut oil use helps prevent hair loss and even stimulates the growth of thinning hair.

I have always had the problem of losing my hair since high school. I am now 37 years old. Since I've been taking the virgin coconut oil for about three months now I no longer lose my hair! It's definitely been a blessing sent by God!
    Jackie

I have also noticed my receding hairline filling in. I have new hair growth and thicker hair since taking virgin coconut oil and massaging with it.
    BKW

Another interesting use for coconut oil is for shaving.

My beard is rather tough...My razor more pulls out the whiskers rather than cuts them, at least that's how it feels. I tried

putting virgin coconut oil on my beard 10 minutes before shaving and it makes a huge difference. I actually shave now. It's great!
James

Deodorant

Body odor, for the most part, is caused by bacteria and fungi feeding off perspiration. The antimicrobial properties of coconut oil prevent the growth of these organisms and help to reduce odor. Because of this, many people use coconut oil as a natural deodorant.

With much ambivalence I tried using coconut oil as a deodorant the past few days. To my surprise it really works! I guess because of the antibacterial properties. Amazing stuff!
Ellie

I tried it about a week ago and it works so well I threw away my roll-on full of chemicals. It doesn't take much and it just soaks right in leaving your skin soft and smooth and a light pleasant coconut scent instead of the chemical scent left by conventional deodorants. I love it! There seems to be no end for the uses of coconut oil.
Valerie

I have been using straight virgin coconut oil as an underarm deodorant since last fall. Works wonders. Works just as good as any antiperspirant/deodorant I have ever used. You just don't have the fragrance from regular deodorant. I have a job that requires a lot of manual labor and my virgin coconut oil deodorant has not failed me yet, even when overheated.
Abigail

Injuries

Coconut oil has an incredible ability to speed healing and reduce pain. Coconut oil can be applied to most any type of injury including cuts, burns, bruises, sprains, insect bites, etc.

Your book Coconut Cures *is very informative and I have learned a lot from it. I have begun using virgin coconut oil and have experienced many health benefits. I also recommend it to others. One of these is a young washer woman. Due to the nature of her work her palms were always cracked and bleeding and her fingers stiff and painful. It was so bad she could hardly move her fingers and thumbs. I advised her to start consuming coconut oil and to apply it on her hands. After only five days her palms stopped bleeding and the most wonderful part is that she can now move her fingers and thumbs without pain.*

W. Yoong

My husband came home with a cut on his hand. Nothing that needed stitches or anything but still a pretty deep cut that had bled quite a bit when it happened. Immediately I ran and got some coconut oil and put it on his cut. He told me when I put it on it was hurting and about ½ hour later it stopped. Two thumbs up for coconut oil again.

Gail

A couple of days ago, my hand got caught in a rope when we were playing tug-of-war with my students. Boy, that hurt! I thought I fractured a bone. Have been waiting for the bruise but it just kept hurting and hurting and hurting, no bruise appeared at all except for the slight bluish, kind of like a discoloration but hardly noticeable on my skin, plus the swelling. I didn't want to apply coconut oil anymore since there was nothing but it started to swell and hurt even more. Applied it before I went to bed, and presto! This morning, swelling has subsided and the pain was just pinch like.

RP

I pinched my thumb badly. It immediately turned purple. It was purple down to the first joint then a little later it swelled. I poured coconut oil in a container and held my thumb in the oil for several minutes. I repeated this procedure a couple of more times

during the day. I couldn't believe it, the next day all of the purple was gone as well as the swelling.
Vonda S

My recent miracle is using coconut oil on the top of my head. I've had a lump on my head for more than 50 years. I must have hit that lump a hundred times, mostly from getting in and out of the car. I began rubbing coconut oil on it several times a day and now it's just a flat place!
RD

Coconut oil possesses the ability to neutralize many poisons or toxins. For this reason, it is useful in treating insect bites. After being bitten massage coconut oil over the infected area. Swelling, inflammation, and pain will greatly subside.

I have been putting coconut oil on my heels, face, and legs sometimes I put it on my neck and shoulders and arms when I go for my walk. The other day I was doing some yard work and noticed something on my legs. I thought it was dirt but it was ants. I quickly turned on the hose and threw off my shoes ands socks fully expecting these ants to be biting and I would be stinging and hurting. I sprayed them off and never felt any bites. I waited a few minutes and to my surprise I had no bites. This just doesn't happen. I had at least 20 ants on each leg not including what was on my shoes and socks. At least twice that, and no bites. The only thing that could have prevented them from biting was coconut oil. I usually hurt several weeks from just one bite and sometimes they leave a scar.
Linda

Regular use of coconut oil can rejuvenate skin tissues and erase scars.

I've been on virgin coconut oil since July and can tell you that I also use it after showering for skin softening. I have a c-section scar that is becoming less noticeable and softer each day.

This is not my first scar (I have four children), but for the others I would use vitamin E without the positive results that the virgin coconut oil is producing now. I am very pleased.
Marcelle

Coconut oil is especially good for soothing and healing burns. I've never seen anything heal burns faster than coconut oil.

My 14 year old granddaughter put some of that chemical hair remover on her legs and got a chemical burn from it. I just put some virgin coconut on her legs and in no time at all it cleared up and no after effects. Wow, there's no end to the wonders of this great stuff.
James

I once poured boiling candles on my finger. It got so red and had a blister. It hurt all day. When I was about to go to sleep, I put the cream (VCO) thickly on top of it and put socks over my hand so that the cream stays on the blister while I am asleep. The next morning, it was not there anymore. No trace at all of the burn.
MB

Natural Sun Screen

One of the oldest uses for coconut oil is as a sun screen/suntan lotion. Islanders have been using coconut oil for this purpose for thousands of years. In the tropics where the climate is hot, islanders traditionally wore little clothing so that they could keep themselves cool. To protect themselves from the burning rays of the hot tropical sun they applied a thin layer of coconut oil over their entire body. This would protect them from sunburn, improve skin tone, and help keep annoying insects away.

Coconut oil was applied on the skin daily. When a mother gave birth one of the first things she would do is to rub coconut oil all over her newborn. Every day coconut oil would be used on the skin. As the children got older they applied the oil themselves. They would continue this practice throughout their lifetime up until the day they died. Many islanders, even today, carry on this practice.

The first commercial suntan and sun screen lotions contained coconut oil as their primary ingredient. Even today many sun screen lotions include coconut oil in their formulas. Coconut oil has an amazing ability to heal the skin and block the damaging effects of UV radiation from the sun. One of the reasons why it is so effective in protecting the skin is its antioxidant properties, which helps prevent burning and oxidative damage that promotes skin cancer.

The first time we went to Hawaii I went to a pharmacy and asked what the locals used for sun block/sunburns. They took me to a generic bottle of coconut oil. I had NEVER had a suntan in my life before that—only burn and peel. With the coconut oil I get a nice tan and no burn. I now have my family all convinced and using it also.
Judy

I burn in the sun easily. I quit using any sunscreens due to toxic ingredients. I read somewhere about using coconut oil on the skin and it will help prevent burning. I tried it yesterday and applied it head to toe. Of course it soaked in immediately and did not feel greasy at all. I can tell you that I normally cannot stay out in the sun all day like that without burning. I gardened in and out of the sun for over eight hours.
FC

Let me tell you about a friend who came with us for an overnight stay on the beach. While bathing on a downcast day (sun was not out), her facial skin became so very red and developed hives. This is one of the cleanest beaches around. So I gave her my ointment made of coconut oil and lavender and I asked her to put it on her face. The next day, it was gone. I asked her to smother a lot of it on her face, neck and extremities the next morning before going into the water; she did and the whole day we were in the ocean, she did not develop any redness/hives/sunburn but had a very even magnificent tan.
MB

84

If you forget to use coconut oil or sunscreen and get a sunburn you can apply the oil on the affected areas to relieve the pain and heal the skin. It works wonders.

[My son] works as a lifeguard at a summer camp for kids (6 and up) and he came home the first day with a sunburn, so we put virgin coconut oil on it and it cleared up overnight.
JA

Eating coconut oil also helps to protect your skin from sunburn. When the oil is consumed the oil fortifies or strengthens the skin so it is more resistant to sunburn. Of course, for best protection you should also apply the oil on the skin as well.

I began eating virgin coconut oil about one and a half years ago. During this time I have completely eliminated all vegetable oils from my diet. In January we moved to the Republic of Panama. Being on the equator I was very curious about how I would react to the sun. I moved from Florida which has intense sun. Here I had previously spent as much as one and a half hours by the pool without sunscreen or lotions. No burn. At the time, my daughter wasn't on virgin coconut oil and went to the beach with 50SPF. Cooked like a French fry in 45 minutes.

This last weekend we took a visitor on a boat trip to a nearby island. They used the 50SPF and my daughter used the 50SPF (now a month on the virgin coconut oil) I used nothing for the day. Our guest burned, we didn't.
RB

I need to add a few words of caution here. Pure virgin coconut oil works exceptionally well as a sunscreen. However, you must be certain it is *pure* virgin coconut oil and not a mixture of coconut oil with other oils, especially polyunsaturated oils such as safflower, soybean, sunflower, or corn oils. These oils, when applied topically will accelerate the damaging effects of UV radiation and quickly burn the skin to a crisp.

Let me tell you about an experience I had. I never use sunscreen. I only use coconut oil and it works beautifully. I have a light complexion and burn very easily. On a hot day I'll get burned if I'm in the sun for more than 30 minutes. If I apply coconut oil on my skin I can stay in the sun five or six hours at a time without reapplying the oil and have no problem with the sun. I've used coconut oil successfully as a sunscreen for many years.

On a recent trip I had the opportunity to go swimming at the beach. I did not have any coconut oil with me and did not want to use commercial sunscreen. I looked for some coconut oil in the local shops and found a dealer selling coconut oil soaps and lotions. To my joy I found a bottle of coconut oil. I looked at the ingredients and it said pure coconut oil and vitamin E, that's it. That sounded good to me, vitamin E is a potent antioxidant it would help protect me from sunburn along with the coconut oil. I purchased it.

When we got to the beach I began applying a generous amount of oil to all the exposed parts of my body. From the very start I noticed something different about the oil. As I rubbed it onto my skin I realized that this oil was not absorbing like virgin coconut oil normally does. It was also much more greasy feeling and pooled on top of my skin. Coconut oil generally absorbs into the body so there is no greasy feel. If you apply too much on a spot you can spread it over more of the skin surface so it all eventually absorbs. But this oil didn't do that. It felt more like a cooking oil.

I was anxious to go out on the beach so I didn't pay much attention to it. I just assumed it must be due to the vitamin E that was added. So I went out in the sun and swam in the water for about 30 minutes and then I began to feel uncomfortable. My skin felt like it was burning. It was strange because this never happened to be before when I used coconut oil. I stayed out another 10 minutes or so until my skin was hurting so much I had to seek shade. Something was not right. My arms, legs, and back were bright red and painful. This was the first sunburn I'd experienced in many years. In fact, I was severely burned, more than I normally would have been for the amount of time I was in the sun.

I knew there was something amiss with the oil I had used. It was very apparent from my reaction and the feel of the oil that it was not pure coconut oil. Apparently, some type of polyunsaturated vegetable oil had been added. This is bad news because polyunsaturated oils will enhance the damage caused by sunburn. I know that some unscrupulous manufacturers will mix coconut oil with cheaper vegetable oils and sell it as virgin coconut oil. Another possibility is that the manufacturer did not use pure vitamin E but used a blend of vitamin E in soybean oil. Vitamin E is generally sold in drug stores and health food stores mixed in a base of soybean oil. It is possible that the manufacturer actually used a soybean based vitamin E mixture and combined that with coconut oil. At any rate, I knew that the oil contained a high percentage of polyunsaturated vegetable oil. This taught me a valuable lesson. I need to know the source of the oil before I use it as a sunscreen.

I tell people all the time they can use coconut oil as a natural sunscreen, but you have to be careful, if you use an impure oil it can cause severe burning. Use only pure virgin coconut oil.

How do you tell if a particular brand of coconut oil is pure? One way is check the melting point. Pure coconut oil melts at 76 degrees F (24 degrees C). At temperatures above this it turns into a liquid. At lower temperatures it becomes solid. If another vegetable oil is mixed into it the melting point will decrease. For example, if the oil in question remains liquid at temperatures much below 76 degrees F you might suspect it has been adulterated. Depending on the room temperature it may take several hours for solid coconut oil to melt or liquid oil to solidify.

You can also compare a known brand of oil with an unknown brand. Put them side by side and leave them together for at least 24 hours. If an oil has been adulterated the difference should be significant. All brands may have some minor differences however.

Another way to tell is to apply several drops of the oil on your arm. Rub the oil in. Coconut oil will absorb into the skin after a few minutes. An adulterated oil will leave a greasy film on the skin that will last for a long time.

Chapter 7

Live Long and Healthy

My Story

Throughout this book you have read numerous success stories from people using virgin coconut oil. I have one more to share with you—my story.

Several years ago I tried a little experiment. In my late 20s I considered myself relatively healthy. I rarely missed a day from work due to illness, although I would go to the office when I wasn't feeling in the best of health. If the illness wasn't too severe, I usually headed off to work. Don't you do the same?

If someone asked me how often I was sick each year, I would think back to the number of days I missed work. It seemed like only two or three, if that many. Somehow, I lost track of all the many days I went to work knowing I was battling some infection. Out of curiosity I decided to conduct an experiment.

I kept a detailed record of every illness I had, whether or not I went to work. If I knew I was fighting an infection or felt one coming on, or experienced allergy-like symptoms I wrote it down. I kept a record of the symptoms, when they started and when they subsided. When I evaluated the record at the end of the year I was shocked. I couldn't believe what I found. It had been a normal year for me healthwise, but I recorded 74 days of illness of one sort or another. This was not the simple aches and pains from everyday life or stress, but definite sickness. I continued this record for six years!

In that time I found that I was sick, on average, for 54.5 days each year! That sounds like a lot but studies by the Centers for Disease Control and Prevention have shown that the average number of sick days each person experiences per year (in the US) is about 65. So I was doing a little better than average. These sick days include major illness as well as minor sniffles, upset stomach, etc. which we all ignore and quickly forget about. If you kept a detailed diary you would be surprised how often you feel "under the weather."

The number of days I was sick surprised me because I was still young and considered myself far healthier than most people. I ate what I felt was a "balanced" diet that included plenty of fruits and vegetables, exercised faithfully an average of four days a week, did not eat many sweets or junk foods. I had always believed in natural heath and tried to live healthfully. So why was I sick so often?

I did eat a lot of vegetable oil, shortening, and margarine. I grew up on these oils because we thought they were healthy. I know better now. Even when I began reducing the total amount of fat and oil in my diet my health didn't seem to improve that much.

I noticed some improvement when I started to eat more fresh fruits and vegetables and made the effort to eliminate convenience and junk foods. The big change, however, occurred when I switched from eating processed vegetable oils and margarine to virgin coconut oil. Since I've been using coconut oil regularly the number of sick days I experience each year has dropped to zero! That's right...no colds, no flus, no stomach aches, no sore throats, no fevers, no allergies, nothing! I haven't been sick for even a single day now in years and I've been around some very sick and contagious people in that time.

Because I use virgin coconut oil almost exclusively in my diet I believe I am protected from many infectious diseases and enjoy improved digestive health—two major benefits of virgin coconut oil. I'm totally free from all chronic degenerative disease. As I write this I'm in my mid-fifties and enjoy better health now than at any time in my adult life. Do the healing properties of virgin coconut oil work? I think so. Why else have I come from 54 days of illness each year, when I was young and supposedly healthy, to none now when I'm middle aged? I've seen many people much younger than I who have died of heart disease, cancer, and other illnesses. With the aid of virgin coconut oil my immune system has been able to fight off every disease-causing germ I have come into contact with over the past several years and kept me free from degenerative disease.

Some people express concern about eating coconut oil because, technically, coconut oil is high in saturated fat. But coconut oil is composed predominately of health promoting medium-chain saturated fats that protect against heart disease. High blood pressure is one of the strongest risk factors associated with heart disease. It's more closely associated with heart disease then high cholesterol. Although I'm in my mid-fifties, because I eat coconut oil I have the blood pressure reading of a 20-year-old (110/60). The average reading of a healthy adult is 120/80. By the time we reach 60 years of age doctors tell us it's typical for blood pressure to increase to 130/90 or more, which is borderline high. As blood pressure increases, cardiovascular health deteriorates and risk of heart disease and stroke increase. Because I eat coconut oil, ten years from now I'll probably still have the cardiovascular health of a 20 year old. Coconut oil protects me from heart disease just as it does Pacific island populations who use it as a part of their everyday diet.

What virgin coconut oil has done for me and for others it can also do for you. You don't need to take my word for it or rely on the testimonies of others. You can prove it for yourself. All you have to do is try it. That's all. Once you begin using the oil you will see changes for the better in your health and your appearance.

Using Virgin Coconut Oil

I suggest that you use virgin coconut oil for all of your cooking needs. For maximum benefit I recommend that you eliminate all other cooking oils from your diet. A little butter or extra virgin olive oil are okay, but do most of your meal preparation with coconut oil.

You can also add virgin coconut oil into your diet by combining it with foods that aren't ordinarily prepared with oil. For instance, you can pour a tablespoon of oil over hot rice, add it to soup, curries, stews, casseroles, and even mix it in hot beverages. There are hundreds of ways to incorporate the oil into your diet. Many people simply take the oil by the spoonful like a dietary supplement. Good quality virgin coconut

90

oil has a mild coconutty flavor and many people enjoy eating it right off the spoon.

People have been trying to eliminate fat from their diets for so long they often don't know how to add fat into their foods. Some find it difficult to incorporate the recommended 2-4 tablespoons of virgin coconut oil into their diets. With this in mind, I've provided a simple way for people to get their allotted amount of coconut oil. I have compiled hundreds of recipes into a book titled the *Coconut Lover's Cookbook*. With this book there is no reason why you can't get the equivalent of 2-4 tablespoons of virgin coconut oil in your diet every day.

I know that virgin coconut oil can make a difference in your life. I've seen it happen in so many others. I would like to hear from you. Write and tell me how coconut oil has affected your life. You can write to me at The Coconut Research Center, P.O. Box 25203, Colorado Springs, CO 80936, USA. For more information about coconut visit my website at www.coconutresearchcenter.org.

Further Study

This book was meant to be a short introduction to the miracles of virgin coconut oil based on the experiences and testimonies of ordinary people like you and me. Because it was brief I only touched on some of health aspects of virgin coconut oil and its uses. There is much more not covered in this book, information on specific illnesses, medical studies confirming its effectiveness, fascinating historical facts, and details on how to use the oil in cooking and body care.

For a more in depth look at the various health aspects of coconut oil I recommend that you read some of my other books on coconut. I have five other books written specifically about coconut. Each is different. Below is a brief description of each.

The Coconut Oil Miracle, 4th Edition*

This is the book that started the coconut oil revolution. Originally published in 2000 this book was the first to reveal the health benefits of coconut oil to the public. It reveals the politics behind the coconut oil smear campaign sponsored by competing industries and how science brought it back into popularity. In this book you will learn why coconut

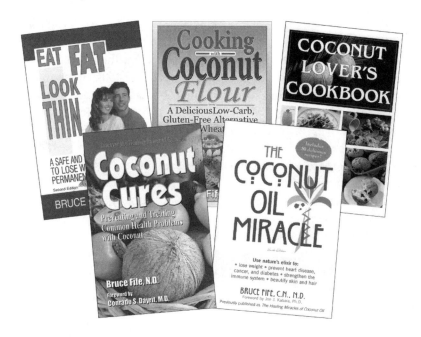

oil is considered the healthiest oil on earth and how it can protect you from heart disease, diabetes, influenza, herpes, Candida, and even HIV.
*Formerly titled *The Healing Miracles of Coconut Oil*

Coconut Cures:
Preventing and Treating Common Health Problems with Coconut
This book reveals the health benefits of the entire coconut—the oil, meat, milk, and water. Discusses in detail why coconut protects against heart disease. Includes an A to Z resource section explaining how to use coconut to treat specific health problems.

Eat Fat, Look Thin:
A Safe and Natural Way to Lose Weight Permanently
This book explains how to use coconut oil to lose excess weight, stimulate metabolism, increase energy, and improve thyroid function. Many people have been able to reduce or even completely eliminate thyroid medication by following the recommendations in this book.

92

Coconut Lover's Cookbook

This book contains 450 recipes using coconut oil, meat, milk, and cream. Recipes include a variety of beverages, salads, soups and stews, curries, main dishes, side dishes, and desserts. Explains how to use coconut oil for cooking and how to get the recommended amount of coconut oil into your diet.

Cooking with Coconut Flour:
A Delicious Low-Carb, Gluten-Free Alternative to Wheat

Coconut flour is made from finely ground coconut meat. It is very high in health promoting dietary fiber and contains no gluten. Coconut flour can be used to make delicious tasting gluten-free breads, cakes, cookies, muffins, and other baked goods. Coconut flour can improve digestion, help regulate blood sugar, protect against diabetes, help prevent heart disease and cancer, and aid in weight loss.

Look for these books in you local health food store or bookstore. If you can't find them in your area go online to www.piccadillybooks.com.

⁂

About the Author

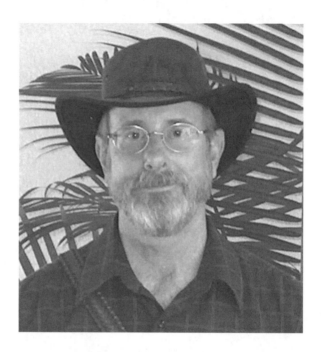

Dr. Bruce Fife, C.N., N.D., is an author, speaker, certified nutritionist, and naturopathic physician. He has written 19 books including *Coconut Cures, The Coconut Oil Miracle* and *Eat Fat, Look Thin.* He is the publisher and editor of the Healthy Ways Newsletter. He serves as the president of the Coconut Research Center (www.coconutresearchcenter.org), a non-profit organization whose purpose is to educate the public about the health and nutritional aspects of coconut.

Dr. Fife was the first one to gather together the medical research on the health benefits of coconut oil and present it in an understandable and readable format for the general public. He is recognized internationally as the world's leading authority on the health aspects of coconut. As such, he travels throughout the world educating medical professionals and laypeople alike on the wonders of coconut. For this reason, he is often referred to as the "Coconut Guru" and many respectfully call him "Dr. Coconut."